I0424908

A Bump in the Road –
My Ride through Roswell Park Cancer Institute

Arthur Paul Reynolds
©2010

All rights reserved. Without limiting the rights under copyright reserved above, no part of this publication may be reproduced, stored in or introduced into a retrieval system, or transmitted, in any form, or by any means (electronic, mechanical, photocopying, recording, or otherwise) without the prior written permission of both the copyright owner and the publisher of this book.

© 2010 by Arthur Paul Reynolds *all rights reserved*

Table of Contents

DEDICATION

This book is dedicated to my wife Carla, and my daughter Collett who stood by me and supported me during this multi-year long adventure. Their positive attitude kept me going and gave me the incentive to get well.

I also dedicate this book to the many doctors, interns, nurses, nurse practitioners, and all the people in the various labs and departments that support the research going on to find a cure for all cancers. I have to especially thank Dr. Fuad Sheriff who first "discovered" I had a problem. If I hadn't kept my appointment that day, and if Dr. Sheriff hadn't noticed that something was wrong, I probably would not be here to write this book.

Finally, I am writing this book for all the people who came before me, all those cancer patients who volunteered for protocols with unknown benefits and side effects. I am writing this for the people who will follow, the hundreds of patients that are still volunteering to participate in the unknown protocols in the belief that they are helping someone else conquer cancer and hopefully, making their journey more successful and less stressful.

I hope this "short story" about my journey helps newly diagnosed leukemia patients understand this disease and know that there is a positive outcome if you believe you can beat this disease. I can't guarantee that everyone who gets leukemia will survive, but perhaps this story will make the journey a little less frightening.

A portion of the sales of this book will be donated to the Roswell Park Cancer Institute.

A copy of this book in e-book format may be found at:

http://www.smashwords.com/books/view/10919

Email your comments/suggestions to:

Paul.publisher@gmail.com

ACKNOWLEDGEMENTS

I want to thank all the people who helped me edit this book. Specifically, Dr. Meir Wetzler, my primary physician at Roswell and Dr. Sharon Cramer, a Professor at Buffalo State College. Their suggestions improved its readability and accuracy. I would especially like to thank all nurses, aides, and support staff; the people in the trenches who where there during the terrible nights of pain and nightmares, who were there when the doctors weren't or couldn't be: Kathy, Lee, Jim, Rick, Patrick, Nancy, Gail, Jodi, Linda, Laura, Jackie, Gwen, Colleen, Zena, Wayne, Karen, Susan, Cheryl, Cathy, Carl, Faj, Lucia, Herbie, William, Angel, and Addie. I hope I have not left anyone out, but know that I really appreciated your support and caring for me while I was in Roswell.

Barbara Anderson, Kim Sweeney, and Kathy Siebold were my bone marrow transplant team. They provided many hours of care-giving and compassion.

I want to thank my primary physicians, Dr. Meir Wetzler, Dr. Maria Baer and Dr. Jim Slack. They gave up a lot of their time to be with the patients in Roswell and when they weren't doing rounds, they were working in their labs to find a cure for leukemia.

I want to thank all of the visiting nurses who gave up their evenings and weekends to come by and check up on me;

and for answering all the questions that Carla and I threw at them.

All the people from Upstate Pharmacy were great in providing my medications; the dedicated group of drivers who delivered my meds in all kinds of weather and with a moment's notice.

I want to mention Dr. Sheriff again, who has kept after me after my treatment, to take better care of myself and for being a good listener during my many visits to his office.

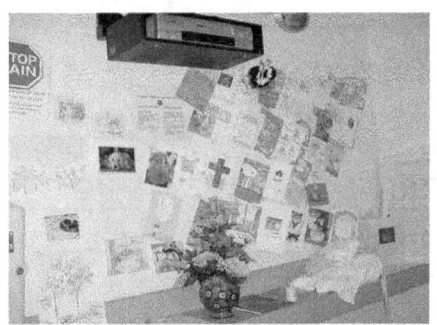 I want to also thank all of the people at Buffalo State College who sent me cards and visited me in Roswell. Knowing that people cared made a difference in my outlook and helped me keep a positive attitude. I want to especially thank Julie Dougherty who donated platelets just specifically for me. Julie said she was afraid the first time she donated her platelets because she wasn't sure what to expect. Her courage helped others decide to donate platelets and as a result, save many lives. Not to lessen Julie's contribution, but to encourage more people to donate, the process is painless (except for the needle stick) and donors get pampered (free lunch, television, etc.) during the process.

PREFACE

During the initial consultations with everyone that came into my hospital room, there was a discussion of what was about to happen to me, and I signed the protocol documents. To this day, I don't remember that conversation, or signing anything. In a later conversation with Dr. Wetzler, he explained that I could have taken one of three paths of treatment as outlined in the diagram below.

Treatment Schema

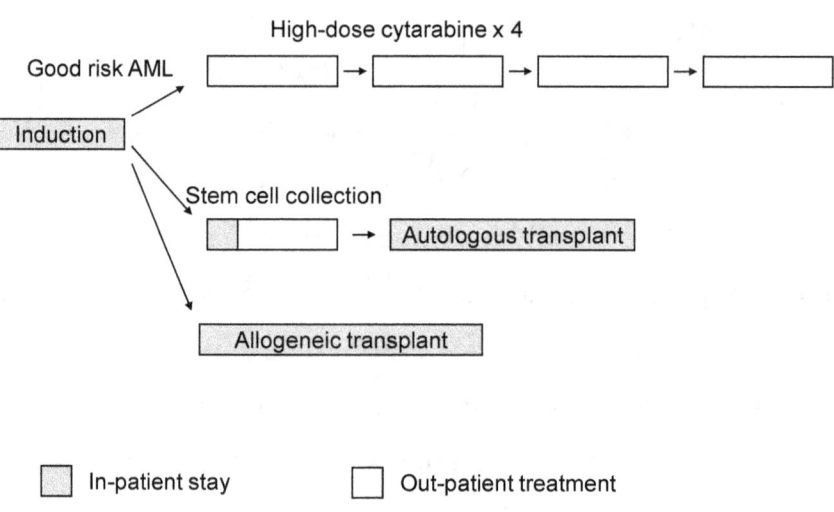

No matter what decision was made, I would have at least one round of chemotherapy known as "Induction". This is the process of initially attempting to kill off the leukemia. If I had "good" leukemia – Good Risk AML, I would be taking the top path.

For any other type of leukemia, I would have to take the middle or bottom path; the difference being, whether or not I could find a compatible stem cell donor. The donor has to match 100% or there is the risk that the transplant would not work, or worse, kill me.

Of course, I had "bad" leukemia – Bad Risk AML; couldn't find a compatible stem cell donor, and ended up taking the middle path.

One thing not shown in the diagram is that there was an additional round of chemotherapy at the end, called IL2 (this is described in the protocol in the appendix). This was an experimental treatment in the protocol at the time and it was an optional, additional treatment. I elected not to have it done. Partly because I had just spent eleven months of my life in and out of Roswell Park Cancer Institute. Secondly, I was tired, physically and mentally, and I didn't think my mind or body would survive another round of harsh chemicals coursing through my system. I just wanted this to be done so I could get on with my life.

In the recent conversation with Dr. Wetzler, there is some indication that having the IL2 procedure lengthens the life span of patients opting for the procedure, and delaying or preventing the return of the leukemia.

When I was a patient, this was unknown territory, but by three or four years out, it was becoming obvious that the IL2 might be beneficial. Since I opted out of this treatment, I will be a "test patient" to see what happens to those who didn't get the IL2. Stay tuned.

INTRODUCTION

It was a dark and stormy night...wait, that's a different story for a different time. Actually it was a very nice afternoon in October 2002 when my adventure really started.

Let me give you some background details. They say things come in threes. My "three" were my parents moving into a new house, my brother-in-law's death, and Leukemia – all within a few days time.

I have a master's degree in educational computing and I decided that a master's degree in library science would be a nice fit. You see, I was getting close enough to retirement to start planning for what I wanted to do when I left my current position. And I had it all planned out. I was going to complete my MLS, buy a motorcycle, retire to New Mexico and get a part time job working in a library. I wanted to live far enough away from the library so it took an hour or so to drive there. I really enjoy riding motorcycles and have had two so far in my life.

On October 14, 2002 my parents called to say they had bought a new house and would be moving in on that weekend. Of course I said I would be home to help them pack and move, but I had already scheduled a doctor's appointment for the following Monday. I said if they really needed me for the weekend, I would cancel my doctor's appointment and be home on Friday. Not necessary they said, there would be

1

enough to do when I got there; and as it turns out it was a good thing I didn't cancel my appointment.

I had been feeling tired and run down, but blamed it on my schedule. I was working a full time job, had a job as an adjunct instructor at a local college and had just started library school. With that schedule, who wouldn't always feel tired and run down? But, I couldn't walk across campus without stopping to catch my breath; and I had to take the elevator instead of the stairs, as I always had, because I just couldn't get up the thirty-nine steps to my office. My mother had congestive heart failure due to a childhood illness and had a valve replaced and I recognized my symptoms as being very similar to hers. That's the reason I finally made an appointment to see my family doctor.

That Friday afternoon, October 18th, my mother called to say my brother-in-law, Rick, aged 47, had just died from a heart attack while driving home from work. My sister was with him and managed to stop the car before it crashed. Well, now I had to go home. But mom said no, wait until there were more details and she would call me back.

She did call back on Saturday and said nothing was going be done until Tuesday or Wednesday because an autopsy had to be done and funeral arrangements were still in the works. I told her I would be home on Monday, right after my doctor's appointment. She said that would be fine. We said our good-byes and hung up the phone - I never made it home to help move or for the funeral.

As you read through this book you will notice that I included dates with some of the narrative. I have done this only when a significant event occurred.

THE STRESS TEST
Monday, October 21, 2002 - 1:00 p.m.

I arrived at the doctor's office at the appointed time and began my physical exam and stress test. I was overweight, had high blood pressure and was just cranky. The stress test began with an EKG and another blood pressure measurement. I had to do this lying down and standing up; I guess these were the baseline measurements. Then I was put on a treadmill and the speed cranked up.

I think I was on the treadmill for less than a minute. I turned very pale; my heart rate shot up to over 200 beats per minute and my blood pressure was off the scale. The doctor quickly stopped the stress test and made me sit down. He said there was something very obviously wrong with me, and he immediately ordered blood work. He was so concerned that he made me wait while the tests were done.

When the results came back he looked very concerned. Apparently a normal, healthy adult has a hemoglobin level of 13-15 g/dL (grams per deciliter); my level was at 6 g/dL. I didn't know it just then, but later my doctor told me I could have passed out and died at any moment. He said I needed to go to the local emergency room where he would set up blood and platelet transfusions for me.

THE EMERGENCY ROOM
Monday, October 21, 2002

I got to the emergency room at about 3:30 p.m. I met with Dr. Walters who was expecting me; and I was moved into one of the "stalls" in the emergency room for my treatment. If you have ever been in an emergency room, you know the rooms are nothing more than areas separated by curtains. One thing I learned about this process is that it can't be rushed. It took 2 to 3 hours for each bag of blood and slightly longer for each bag of platelets to be transfused. Carla, my wife, was by my side the whole time. I convinced her it was okay to leave for a while to get something to eat and that I would be OK. Around 11:00 p.m., I was able to get her to go home to try to sleep. I told her that I would call if anything changed. If I had to, I could take a taxi home.

I think I received at least two pints of blood and two bags of platelets. The whole process dragged on until 6:00 a.m. Tuesday morning. I was not able to sleep much, as people were constantly coming and going, I was moved to a different bed twice; there was nothing to eat and going to the bathroom with the transfusion/infusion stand attached to me was an adventure in itself.

Tuesday, October 22, 2002

Around 7:30 a.m., Dr. Walters came in with another doctor who he introduced as Dr. Hong – an oncologist/hematology specialist. Even with my limited knowledge of medicine and being extremely tired, I was able to figure he was a blood cancer doctor. A thousand things ran through my mind, but I tried to remain calm.

Dr. Hong was pleasant enough as he explained that there was something wrong with my blood. Too many white cells, not enough red cells, and more testing would have to be done. He said they had made plans to move me to Roswell Park Cancer Institute in Buffalo, New York. I was stunned; I wanted to cry -- I wanted to scream; this couldn't be happening to me. Why me, why now?

I was able to call Carla, who was sleeping and sounded groggy when she answered the phone. I tried to tell her what was going on without scaring her. She managed to get dressed and get to the hospital just as they were preparing to take me out to the ambulance for the ride to Roswell. I can still remember the look in her eyes – panic, fear, questions, and more. It was all I could do to keep from crying. I had just a minute to give her a hug and a kiss before I was placed on the gurney and taken out to the ambulance.

I had never been in an ambulance before, so I detached myself from my condition and found the ride to be rather interesting. The medics were quite friendly and answered all my questions. The trip took about twenty minutes and at the end of it I was wheeled into the lobby of Roswell. That made wonder how they could have just spent several million dollars

remodeling Roswell Park Cancer Institute and no one thought
of building an emergency room or an emergency entrance to
the hospital. So I was wheeled in through the lobby where I
was unloaded into a chair to wait further instructions.

Carla and I got through the admitting paperwork and
we walked back to the seating area to wait because there were
no beds available for me. We waited almost an hour and I was
finally told I could go up to Five West. We grabbed the nearest
elevator and rode up to the fifth floor; neither one of us said
much of anything. We had no clue about what was going to
happen over the next few days – I never imagined that the
elevator ride would lead me into a place wherein I would lose
almost a year of my life.

I decided to keep a journal because I knew I would
never remember all of this. You are reading my story, taken
from the notes in my journal. In fact, Roswell encourages this
process. One of the first things I received after arriving in the
hospital was a small journal entitled, "TO WRITE, TO DRAW,
TO DREAM"; which consisted of many blank pages,
inspirational sayings, and quotes from people who have
survived cancer. I believe it was supplied by the Leukemia and
Lymphoma Society. They encouraged patients to write about
their experiences and provided this starter journal.

At the bottom of the first page are these inspirational
words; "We hope that this book will be a useful outlet for you

while you visit the Roswell Park Cancer Institute. If you have ideas on how people can use this, let us know." I liked the idea that I was here just for a "visit".

Since we didn't know what was going to happen over the next few days we didn't tell our daughter, Collett, what was going on. She was going to school at SUNY Geneseo and we didn't want to add to her stress level. Once I was admitted, Collett did come home on the weekend for a quick visit.

THE ADVENTURE BEGINS
Tuesday, October 22, 2002 – Later in the day

We arrived on the fifth floor, west wing; I went to the admitting desk, gave them my paperwork and was escorted into my room. Little did I know that I would not leave the hospital for five weeks! I can't imagine how a single person (or someone with no immediate family) would handle this situation. I was scared, concerned about my wife, my daughter, my job, and my house. Would I ever go home again?

The situation wasn't made much better in the next few hours. During that time the following things happened: a social worker stopped by to tell me she would do everything she could to be sure I wouldn't lose my house or my job. A patient advocate came around to let me know he was there to help with any issues I might have during my "stay" at Roswell. The protocol nurse on my case, Kim Sweeney, explained my protocol; and had me sign what seemed like a hundred documents. She told me that everything being done was voluntary and I could leave any time I wanted to (a copy of the protocol is in the appendix and I honestly don't remember signing it). Finally, the team of doctors that would be working on my case, Dr. Meir Wetzler, Dr. Maria Baer, and Dr. Jim Slack, dropped by with a gaggle of students (nurses, nurse practitioners, and interns) to introduce themselves and to give me an overview of what to expect for the next thirty to forty days.

I was still trying to digest the fact that I was in Roswell Park Cancer Institute, that I had cancer (of some sort), and my life would never be the same.

I am really glad that Carla was there, because she was more focused than I, she **really heard** what the doctors where saying. I was just so overwhelmed that when someone new came in, and started talking, it was like one of those "Charlie Brown" cartoons where the teacher is talking and it's just, "Whaa whaa whaa whaa." During the whole process, if something major was going on and Carla was there, she took notes. Each day she would review with me what the doctors actually said. I was still in a state of denial, and couldn't remember a lot of what the doctors said. They explained things very quickly, and used a lot of medical jargon. That's one reason for me starting a journal; I would attempt to record events as they happened so I could review them later.

Understand now, that at this point Carla and I have had nothing to eat or drink since 6:00 a.m. We're both tired, I'm feeling cruddy because it's been over 48 hours since I've taken a shower, I am scared for my wife and what she is thinking, and I was just told I am not going home for five or six weeks. It was just so overwhelming -- I was in shock and couldn't react to any of this. Also, I had not been able to communicate with work to let them know I was not coming in, nor had I had any contact with my daughter, parents or sister.

So the routine began. I got out of my street clothes, put on one of those ridiculous hospital gowns and got into my bed. I had more blood work done, more blood pressures taken; I was examined from head to foot. I was sent to radiology where I had everything x-rayed; I received my first MUG-A exam[1]. I was being checked out to see if I was in good enough shape to survive the treatment I was about to receive. As they say, sometimes the cure is worse than the disease.

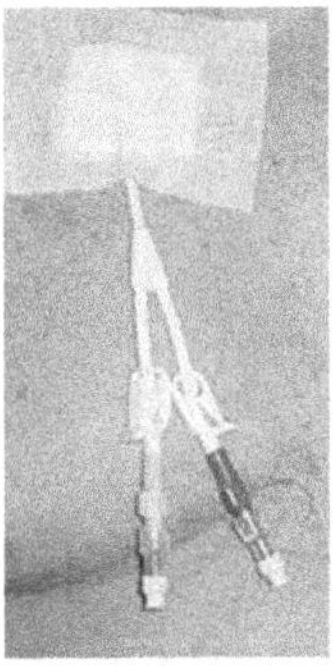

Figure 1 Hickman Catheter

I was taken to another part of the hospital where a medical port – a Hickman Line or Catheter - was inserted in my chest into my jugular vein. It had two "ports" attached (one red, one blue) where medications could be injected. This was done to save the veins in my arms and legs and cut down on the pain I was going to experience. These ports would be used to draw blood, inject the chemotherapy, and any other medications I might need during my stay.

It's now about 5:30 - 6:00 p.m. Carla is with me and I finally settle down in my room and someone brought in supper for both Carla and me. One thing I can say about Roswell is that they have the best food of any hospital I have ever been in. It was almost as good as the food at some of the local restaurants.

---

[1] This consists of getting a radioactive injection and then laying a special x-ray machine for twenty minutes to have hundreds of pictures of my heart taken and reviewed.

All of this would be lost on me when the chemo started working in a few days.

I could tell Carla was tired and worried, and she needed to go home. I didn't want her to leave because I was worried about her state of mind; but I convinced her she needed to get some rest and she left around 9:30 p.m. I am pretty sure she didn't sleep much that first night, or any night during that first round, but at least she was at home in comfortable surroundings.

I was concerned about my family more than myself. I knew I was in good hands and would receive good care. Carla, a lawyer specializing in elder law, and working full time; how was she going to cope with worrying about me, her job, the house and our daughter Collett?

All of this happened so fast that Collett wasn't aware that I was in the hospital, let alone sick. She was in her second year at SUNY Geneseo and working at the Target Store in Rochester, New York. Collett had a friend there named Brett Pirdy. He was going to Rochester Institute of Technology and worked with Collett at the Target store. They were pretty close and were dating. Brett's mother lived close by and the two of them would travel home most weekends to visit. His mother was not in the best of health either, so he would spend a lot of time visiting her and helping out as much as he could.

DAY TWO
Wednesday, October 22, 2002 – about 7:30 a.m.

The only thing I remember from the night before was the nurses coming in every four hours or so to take my "vitals" and to make sure I was okay (to this day I cannot sleep more than four hours at a time without waking up). The bed I was on used an air mattress instead of a regular mattress and had an automatic inflation system on it. Every time I moved the pump would come on and inflate the area I just moved from, as you can imagine, this took some getting used to.

Around 9:00 a.m. Dr. Wetzler came into my room to give me some details about what was going to happen over the next few weeks. He said that they couldn't tell what kind of leukemia I had from just the blood work and that they would have to do a bone marrow biopsy.

There are four types of leukemia in two categories: Acute and Chronic. These are outlined on the next page.

Acute Myelogenous Leukemia (AML) and **Chronic Myelogenous Leukemia** (CML)

AML, also known as acute myelogenous leukemia, is a cancer of the myeloid line of white blood cells, characterized by the rapid proliferation of abnormal cells which accumulate in the bone marrow and interfere with the production of normal blood cells.

AML is the most common acute leukemia affecting adults, and its incidence increases with age. Although AML is a relatively rare disease, accounting for approximately 1.2% of cancer deaths in the United States, its incidence is expected to increase as the population ages.

Acute Lymphocytic Leukemia (ALL) and **Chronic Lymphocytic Leukemia** (CLL)

ALL, also known as acute lymphocratic leukemia, causes damage and death by crowding out normal cells in the bone marrow, and by spreading (metastasizing) to other organs. ALL is most common in childhood and young adulthood with a peak incidence at 4-5 years of age, and another peak in old age.

They are called acute because the symptoms appear relatively quickly and the disease needs to be treated right away. The symptoms for the chronic type appear over a period of time and can be mistaken for other illnesses. Once diagnosed however, the treatment also needs to be done quickly. The medicines used for the two varieties are slightly different.

Later that day, Dr. Baer and an intern came to my room to take a biopsy (the first of many). There was a nurse there to assist, and to collect the samples. The doctor asked me if I wanted to be awake for the procedure or to get a conscious sedation[2]. Keeping with the macho theme, I decided to go au natural and stay awake. It took four or five biopsies before it sunk in that "conscious sedation" was the way to go. I tended to babble a lot while sedated -- I wonder if I incriminated myself in any way?

To get a sample of my bone marrow, the doctor uses a special tool that first punctures the skin and bone. This is basically a sharp, large bore needle that has to be pressed and twisted to get through the skin and break through the bone. Once this is done, another tool (similar to a corkscrew) is inserted into this tube and twisted. As it turns, it brings the bone marrow up with it and the marrow is placed into a test tube and sent off to the lab. The doctor's preferred spot for getting bone marrow is from the hip, about where a belt would sit.

During the process the doctor must have hit one of my nerves because all of a sudden my legs went stiff and I felt a shooting pain go all the way up my back. This scared the doctor and she kept saying, "I'm so sorry." The whole process took only five or ten minutes but seem a lot longer than that.

---

[2] Conscious sedation is a light, general anesthesia that dulls the pain, but allows you to stay awake and be aware of your surroundings.

The doctor, intern and nurse left after that, and I spent most of that day just waiting for test results, and getting used to my new "home". Carla had come to visit in time to see the procedure and was bothered by it. We spent the rest of that day alternating between just talking about what was going to happen and watching TV. She left to get supper in the cafeteria -- later we learned she could order supper and have it delivered with mine so we could eat meals together in my room.

When I was admitted I received a "green card" that had all my important information on it. This also allowed Carla to get a discount on parking in the ramp near the hospital.

My chemo couldn't start until it was determined exactly what type of leukemia I had. To while away the time, I was given a handbook to read, to understand what I would be going through. On page 17 of the handbook it says that children between 2 and 10 years old have a 40% chance for a cure. I had access to the Internet and decided to check out options for a person my age. According to several sites on the Internet, the percentage for recovery and/or remission gets worse as a patient gets older, over 60 years of age, the outlook was pretty grim. Having access to the Internet to do research is wonderful, but sometimes the information provided can be depressing.

DAY THREE
Wednesday, October 23, 2002

I think it was around 9:00 a.m. when Dr. Wetzler came in to tell me that they hadn't been able to get a good enough sample of bone marrow to determine which kind of leukemia I had. They would have to do another biopsy to get a better sample.

Later that day, Dr. Baer came for the next sample. This time she took it out of my left hipbone. I found out later that my right hipbone provided a better sample and was easier to get to. From that point on, all my biopsies were taken from my right side. Seven years later I still have a small scar in the pattern of little circles on my lower right side; it has its value as I can always tell you when the weather will change.

The rest of the day passed quietly. I was able to eat and watch TV. Later, Carla came in and brought some pajamas, and mail from home. We ate supper and watched a little TV together. It was easy to tell that Carla was not getting enough sleep; after we ate she curled up in the chair, and took a nap.

ROUND ONE BEGINS
Thursday, October 24, 2002

When Carla came in, she brought some of my clothes from home so I didn't have to wear those silly gowns provided by the hospital. I switched to pajamas later on because the room was either too hot or too cold and there never was an in-between.

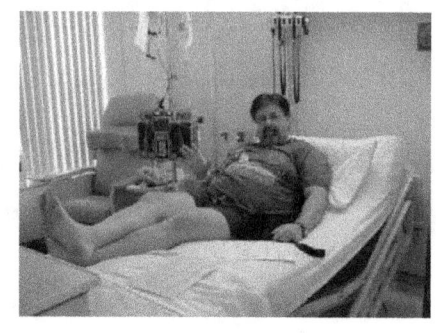

Figure 2 Paul receiving chemo

While I waited for everything to start, I was placed on fluids. In the picture above you can see my medical pump. This pole would become my buddy and I named it "Barney" (after one of my favorite cartoon characters – Barney Rubble). We would be inseparable for the next five weeks. Also, notice the hair. It was never to be like that again.

Kim Sweeney, the research nurse in charge of my protocol, explained that I had three options: (1) Do nothing -- just have support, come to the hospital for routine checkups and infusions; (2) go for standard treatment; or (3) go for special experimental treatment. I told her I would go for one of the last two treatment options[3]. Going with the first option basically meant that I was going to die.

---

[3] Which option that was ultimately selected would be determined by the kind of leukemia I had.

The blood work and bone marrow biopsy determined that I didn't have the "good" leukemia, so I had to follow a standard protocol for my treatment. Apparently, there is some kind of lottery system because I was told that the computer didn't pick me for an experimental treatment. So I was "stuck" with the standard, proven treatment.

The Chemo Infusion

What I didn't realize was that getting the chemotherapy was relatively easy; it was the delay that knocked me out. After the port was in place, the nurses simply hung a bag of the chemo drugs on the stand and connected it to one of my ports.

The chemotherapy drugs for the first round are infused twenty-four hours a day, for seven days. After seven days all the chemo was stopped, but the various fluids continued to be infused. On about day fourteen I found out what chemo was all about. It seems that it takes a week or so after the infusions stop before the chemo actually takes effect. That's when the nausea, diarrhea, mucusitis, and pain start to be noticed.

For the first week I thought, "This isn't bad." I was eating really well. The dietician would stop by with her meal plans, and I planned out my meals for the first two or three weeks – pizza, chicken, beef wellington, pudding, pie, coffee, and a variety of juices. On day nine or ten, I think I planned on eating chicken ala king. The first bite was okay. After that, it tasted like rubber and glass at the same time. It hurt to chew and it hurt to swallow; and the smell of the food was causing me to be nauseous. Some days were better than others, and I was able to eat. Some days were really bad, and I settled for Jell-O and hot tea.

The nurses said I would not want to drink coffee after a while: of course I didn't believe them. Before I went into Roswell, I was drinking two pots of coffee a day. The second or third day after the chemo hit, I stopped drinking coffee completely. It was to be hot tea only. I couldn't even put honey in the tea because the "bee spit" that is used to make honey contained too many germs and I didn't have an immune system anymore.

The chemo messed with everything, including my digestive system. I switched between diarrhea and constipation. There is no privacy in any hospital, but is seemed that whenever I needed to go to the bathroom, one of the nurses or doctors would need to see me for something. I started getting nervous about being in the bathroom for anything. By the way, everything, and I mean everything, was measured while I was in the hospital. All my intakes and outputs were measured on an hourly basis. If my output didn't match my input, I was put on lasix (a loop diuretic, a water pill that prevents your body from absorbing too much salt, allowing the salt to instead be passed in your urine) for a few days. It's called lasix because its effects last for six hours, and it is very effective.

Once I knew that I was going to be in the hospital for a while and I knew I was going to be semi-mobile, I had Carla bring in my laptop computer. I started creating a website that detailed all the things that were happening to me. I think this helped my mental state a little; it surely helped me keep track of everything. I was also able to keep in touch with people through my work email; just having some contact with the outside world helped me keep a positive attitude about this "trip".

My website is located at:

http://sites.google.com/site/paulreynoldsproject/

Monday, November 4, 2002

It's interesting how people mark important events. I imagine that most people who were alive when President Kennedy was killed, still remember where they were and what they were doing (I was in seventh grade French class). Roswell became a time marker for us. We started talking about dates Before Cancer (BC). Today, we celebrate Collett's 20th birthday in Roswell. Carla brought in some small gifts and the nurses ordered a special birthday tray for Collett. It came with a cupcake with a candle in it. It was special because I was still here to see it, and it was special because we could all be together. I wasn't sure if I would see anymore of her birthdays, or mine for that matter, but I was going to give it my best shot.

Sunday, November 10, 2002

The chemo messes with everything, so I'm not sure I have my dates and times correct, even though I tried to write in my journal as soon as something significant happened.

According to my count it is now Day 13 in the hospital and Day 11 after the chemo infusion was completed. Even though this is tough on my mind and body, I have a lot of people here who seem to care about me and they are looking out for my best interests.

I worry about Carla because she has to go home and take care of everything: the house, the cat, her job, and Collett. People don't realize that having cancer is possibly worse for the family than the person going through treatment. Of course, the patient is going through a lot of physical pain and mental anguish, but there is twenty-four hour support. If the smallest thing happens, there are several people there in a minute to help. The family is home dealing with daily issues and worrying about the family member in the hospital. There is not always someone to come to the immediate aid of the family members at home.

Tuesday, November 12, 2002

I had another bone marrow biopsy today. This biopsy went better than the other two. It takes a few days to get the results from the lab, but the doctors always let me know what's happening.

My Hair

Another myth about chemo is that it makes your hair fall out right away. My hair stayed attached until almost the end of the first round. I was running my hand through my hair one day and noticed that it was

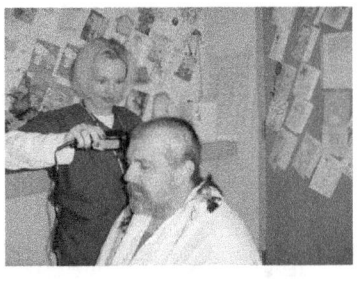

Figure 3 Jodi cuts Paul's hair

starting to come out. So, instead of having it come out in clumps and looking silly, Jodi, one of the nurses, shaved my head. That in itself was a harrowing experience since I was the first patient that she had shaved. She came at me with the wrong edge of the electric razor and I thought for sure I was going to lose an ear, or at least be scarred for life.

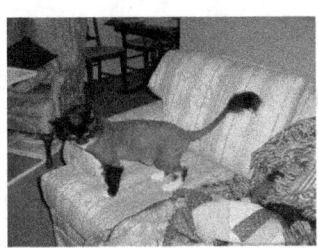

I mentioned our cat earlier. His name was BO, which stood for Body Odor. I named him that because we got him from the SPCA and he would let out

Figure 4 BO after his haircut   the stinkiest farts -- even worse than some people I know. He also had a skin condition that made him smelly at times. He was Carla's constant companion while I was in the hospital and seemed to sense she needed some company and comforting.

23

He had a skin condition that the vets could not diagnose. So, once every six months he would go to the vets for a shave and a special bath. One of his treatments coincided with me losing my hair and I posted his picture on my website. Unexpectedly, we had a lot in common.

I got all kinds of emails as a result of posting the picture, most people understood, but some wanted to know why I was so mean to my cat. I tried to explain that the cat was shaved due to health concerns. But some people just didn't want to hear it.

Monday, November 18, 2002

I survived another night without spiking a temperature. Dr. Wetzler said that if I stay fever-free he would let me go home tomorrow. He also said there's no reason to keep my catheter, so that will come out before I go home. I'm so excited. It's like when I was a kid and it is Christmas Eve. Getting discharged from the hospital was almost as bad as getting discharged from the Army (I spent three years in the Army).

Even though I was going home and would be home for the holidays, I would still have to come back to Roswell twice a week for blood tests, infusions and other checkups. The doctors wanted to make sure I didn't relapse between rounds.

Since I was just discharged from Roswell and my immune system was nonexistent, I wasn't allowed to have visitors, so no company for Thanksgiving this year. But this was still one of the best Thanksgivings I have ever had.

END OF ROUND ONE
At Home
Monday, December 2, 2002

I have been home for a while and am awaiting word from Dr. Wetzler on what to do. At this point, I was going back to Roswell every few days for check-ups, blood work, and infusions. The last I heard was that I was supposed to return to Roswell on December 12 to start Round Two of my treatment, with the actual infusion starting on December 17. This means I would have to spend Christmas and New Year's in the hospital. This was not a pleasant thought.

Dr. Wetzler called a couple of days later to tell me that my protocol nurse, Kim Sweeney (the doctor called her the "protocol police") said the 17th was too soon to start my second round of chemo. I would have to wait at least two weeks before starting my second round of chemo. This meant I could enjoy the holidays at home.

At this same time, Dr. Wetzler said I should be looking for a bone marrow donor and suggested I talk to my family. My sister Janine was the most likely candidate since my mother was too old and not in the best of health. So Carla and I made a trip to Roswell's business department to get the paperwork started to see if Jan could be my donor. This process would take a few weeks, so my second round of chemo was set for

January 6, 2003. There was some concern about the length of time between the rounds of chemo; there was a small chance I could relapse during this period.

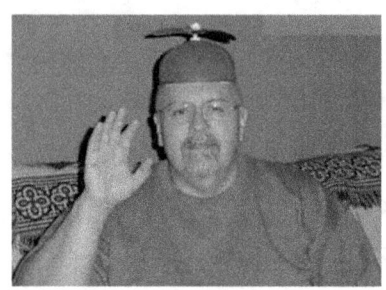

I was feeling a little down and needed something to cheer me up. Some people from my office sent me a surprise gift and it came at just the right time. I threatened to

Figure 5 Paul at home

wear it to work, but Carla wouldn't let me out of the house with it on.

Bone Marrow Donor

Friday, December 27, 2002

Barbara Anderson, the bone marrow transplant coordinator, called to say my sister could not be a donor. The blood tests showed that she was only a 50% match for me. (I asked my mother which one of us was adopted – since my sister was only 50% compatible, she or I must have been adopted. My mother didn't see the humor in my comments.) I could still attempt to do an allogeneic (donor) transplant or go for an autologous (auto) transplant.

The concerns were that if I go with the allogeneic transplant, I could run the risk of the donor's white cells attacking my cells as "foreign bodies" and actually attacking my organs. This is called Graft-vs.-Host-Disease. Also, if this did happen (or the transplant failed), I would have no recourse. If I elected to go with the autologous transplant and it failed, I could still try the donor option. The concern about an auto transplant is that there is the risk of relapse. The success of the transplant depends on the health and age of the patient. At 52 years old, I was considered young.

Monday, December 30, 2002

The holidays went by without issues, but I developed a cough and it scared me. I wasn't sure if it was a cold or not; if it was, what would that do to my treatment? So, Carla drove me into Roswell and I underwent some tests. My lungs were clear and, although low, my counts were okay.

After the New Year, both Carla and I got sick with something. Carla had it worse than I did, but it passed in a couple of days. I was tired and slept most of the time for the next few days.

Friday, January 3, 2003

I'm getting ready to head back to Roswell to start round two: consolidation. For some reason I felt very apprehensive about this round; I don't know why, but I suppose since I now know what's going to happen, I wasn't too excited about going through it again.

The chemo causes all sorts of side effects. I was given some drugs to lessen the effects. Of course, some of those drugs had their own side effects, so I had to take more drugs to offset those effects. On the next page is a list of what I was taking.

Levaquin -

a quinolone antibiotic used in adults as a lung, sinus, skin, and urinary tract infection treatment

Acyclovir -

commonly used antiviral drug

Metoclopramide -

used short-term to treat heartburn caused by gastro esophageal reflux

Diflucan -

used to treat and prevent fungal infections

Proton x -

manages erosive acid reflux, treat associated symptoms of acid reflux, and heal esophageal erosions

Docusate -

is given to make stools softer and easier to pass

Oxydocone -

opioid pain reliever

Vancomycin -

reduce the development of drug-resistant bacteria and maintain the effectiveness of Vancomycin and other antibacterial drugs

Sodium Chloride Spray -

for dry eyes

Triamcinolone Cream -

used to treat allergies, skin conditions, ulcerative colitis, and arthritis

Dexamethasone -

a potent synthetic member of the glucocorticoid class of steroid hormones. It acts as an anti-inflammatory and immunosuppressant

ROUND TWO BEGINS
Monday, January 6, 2003

Carla and I arrived at Roswell at 8:30 a.m. to admit me for Round Two, consolidation. After having a few weeks off to recover from the first round of chemo, this round is supposed to completely kill off any leukemia left and prepare me for growing my own, healthy stem cells. These cells will be infused into me after the third round of chemo. I was admitted to five-west again, but this time I had a room with no view. Not that this was important, since as soon as the effects of the chemo hit, a good view was the least of my concerns.

This time around I had a new Hickman two-lumen catheter inserted. This device was supposed to be inserted into my left chest since my first one was in my right side. The doctors tried to vary things so no one part of my body was over stressed. Just my luck, though, the veins in my left side were occluded so the new port had to be put in my right side. It was inserted directly into my jugular vein. Because they first tried the left side and finally ended up using my right side, both sides of my chest were really sore. It hurt this time to have the port inserted.

I went back to my room to start another week of chemo. This time I am getting Ara-C (Ara-C is one of the older chemotherapy drugs which have been around and in use for many years. Ara-C is a clear, colorless liquid given by intravenous route) and Etoposide VP-16 (Etoposide is a colorless fluid. It is also available as pale pink capsules).

Receiving chemotherapy is not a hard or painful process. What most people don't understand is that the side effects of chemo are what cause all the problems and the side effects don't usually manifest themselves until several days after the chemo is stopped being infused.

Unlike the first round of chemo, the drugs for this round were given in doses. This round started at 9:30 p.m. and would be infused in four doses. In this round the side effects showed up quicker than during the first round. My appetite is almost gone; food looks good, but there is no flavor. The nausea is back with a vengeance; the smell of food triggered my gag reflexes almost immediately. Also, the mucusitis is back, making it difficult to chew and swallow my food; even Jell-O is hard to eat. The chemo drugs affected my eyes; it made them photophobic[4].

Several more drugs were added to counteract these symptoms:

Zophram -	for the nausea
Phenergran -	used to treat allergy symptoms and prevent motion sickness
Atavan -	a benzodiazepine used to treat anxiety disorders or anxiety associated with depression
Oxydocone -	an opioid analgesic medication synthesized from thebaine (a minor constituent of opium).

---

[4] This is when the eyes are very sensitive to light.

Friday, January 10, 2003

This round of chemo caused severe leg cramps, and pain all over my body. I also developed a deep-red rash over most of my body. I started taking morphine for the leg cramps and a fentanyl patch (one of the most powerful opioid analgesics with a potency approximately 81 times that of morphine) on my arm.

After talking to the doctor and nurses, it seems it's more likely that the growth hormone shots caused the "bone ache" I was experiencing. It got to the point where it was hard to sit or lay down for any length of time. Walking seemed to help the ache go away, but that lasted for only a short time. Between the nurses' encouragement and the bone ache, I was certainly getting a lot of exercise walking around the ward.

I found the best way to get any rest was to sleep in the recliner in my room. But it seemed that just as I got comfortable and started falling asleep, a nurse or an aide came in to take my vitals, give me meds, or to just check up on me.

Another side effect of the chemo and other drugs was constipation or diarrhea. For some people, it's constipation, for others, it's diarrhea. For me, it was constipation (thus the docusate – a stool softener).

Saturday, January 11, 2003

I am anticipating going home to recover from this round of chemo, but during the night I spiked a fever of 39^0 C or about

105^0 F. If I have a fever, I can't go home. Dr. Wetzler decided I needed to stay until Sunday. He wanted to watch my rash and keep an eye on my fever.

The doctors and nurses encouraged patients to walk around the ward. The ward was arranged with the nurses' station set up as an island in the middle of the floor with the rooms around the outside. Twenty times around this loop is about 1/8 of a mile. When I was feeling anxious or bored, I would grab my IV stand, "Barney", and do the loop. I must have walked 15 or 20 miles while I was there.

Sunday, January 12, 2003

I was waiting for Dr. Wetzler to come by to let me know if I was going home today or not. I tried to eat my breakfast while I was waiting, but the chemo has totally destroyed any sense of taste that I had had; I can't even make spit. Everything tasted bland, but sweet at the same time. No amount of salt seemed to get rid of the sweet tastes.

I think just the thought that I might go home today made me feel better. If I did have to stay, I was getting a shower. It had been almost a week since my last one. But, it was my lucky day and around 2:00 p.m., the doctor said I could go home.

END OF ROUND TWO
Back Home
Monday, January 13, 2003

The doctor let me come home yesterday. After dealing with the paperwork and packing up all my things, I got home about 3:00 p.m. All I wanted to do was sleep. I set up my place on the couch, got my favorite blanket and hat and settled in. Chemo has made me constantly sleepy and cold. I used to sit around in shorts and a T-shirt, even in the winter. Now I have to wear a sweat suit, socks and a hat to even begin warming up. I usually added a down comforter too. I just couldn't get warm.

Around 3:30 p.m. Upstate Pharmacy delivered my lifetime supply of vancomycin. Right behind the delivery guy, the visiting nurse from Univera showed up to show me how to infuse the drug. The vanco comes in little pressurized balls, pretty neat actually. I simply cleaned my ports with a saline solution and heparin (a highly-sulfated glycosaminoglygan – pharmaceutical grade heparin is derived from mucosal tissues of slaughtered meat animals, such as pig intestine or cow lung) and connected one of the balls to one of the lines and carried on as usual. It took about an hour to infuse one dose and I had to do this once every 12 hours.

Tuesday, January 14, 2003

Being an outpatient means that I still had to visit Roswell two or three times a week. So, at 8:30 a.m. on Tuesday the 14th I'm back in Roswell for blood work and a check on my

33

antibiotics. I don't know how Carla did it, but she always managed to be available to take me to Roswell. My life was disrupted and I was away from work, but Carla missed a lot of work too. People don't understand how much a disease like leukemia (or any cancer) and its treatment disrupts everything for everyone, not just the patient.

The vanco infusion was changed to every eight hours instead of 12, which means I had to get up in the middle of the night to infuse the stuff. It is said that a lot of rest helps recovery. Well, there wasn't a lot of rest, either at home or in the hospital.

The Univera visiting nurse stopped by to show Carla and me how to change the dressing that covers my port. (Yes, I went home with the second port still imbedded in my chest, but this is a good thing because otherwise I would have to stick myself with a needle several times a day.) The dressing has to be changed every time I take a shower. At home, I could do this every couple of days; at the hospital, a shower was a once a week treat. I'll tell you, a nice hot shower never felt so good in my life.

Because I wasn't as good a boy as I should have been, I had issues with my fluid intake. It was decided that I needed to infuse myself with a saline solution. The visiting nurse showed Carla and me how to install the fluid bag into the pump, how to turn on/reset the pump, and how to hook up all the tubes. So now, "Barney junior" was at home with me, following me around the house. Our house is a split-level configuration, so it was interesting trying to get the pump from one room to another, up and down stairs, through narrow doorways, etc.

Thursday, January 16, 2003

I had a 7:30 a.m. appointment in the infusion clinic today. It was a good thing too. I felt like I was run over by a truck. As it turns out, I didn't eat enough or take in enough fluids. I was diagnosed with pancreatitis (an inflammation of the pancreas) and readmitted to Roswell around 3:00 p.m. I was admitted to Five West and everyone was surprised to see me back so soon. Fluid intake is very important, almost more important than eating. I was put on "NPO" (nothing by mouth), hooked up to fluids, antibiotics and painkillers. I think because I couldn't eat anything, I really wanted ice cream. I realized (only now) that had I eaten better and taken in more fluids while I was home, I wouldn't be in my current situation.

Sunday, January 19, 2003

Still in Roswell, but since today was a dressing change day, I got to take a nice long shower. The water in Roswell never got hot, so I had a nice long, tepid shower, but it still felt *so good*. My vitals are not good enough for me to go home yet, so it looks like birthday number 53 will be celebrated in Roswell.

A new doctor, Dr. Jim Slack, stopped by to explain that my pancreas was putting out large doses of a digestive enzyme (even though I wasn't eating) and that was what was causing all my pain. The enzymes help digest the food I ate. Normally, these enzymes don't become active until they reach the small intestines. Since I have been pain free for a day or two, I can now start on a clear liquid diet – Jell-O, water, tea, juice, etc.

When I was readmitted, Carla had a chance to get a free mammogram while she was waiting for me to be processed. She was told they found "something" and she would have to be reexamined. Both of us were discouraged since she already had enough on her mind.

All the fluids and drugs gave me diarrhea so I am taking Imodium to fight that. It seems to be working. It amazed me how one drug can fix things, but comes with so many side effects that it seems better to deal with the initial problem without them.

A new nurse, Rich, was on the floor today. I called him "mother hen" because he seemed so concerned about my well-being. He stopped in every hour or so to make sure everything was okay; he took special care when cleaning my ports.

The bilirubin count in my liver is at a "high normal"; this causes jaundice, making the whites of my eyes turn yellowish and my skin look like I'm tanned. So that has to be watched, and was probably caused by the "stress" of fasting due to my pancreatitis. It should clear up on its own once my pancreas gets back to normal. Special treat today, I got to have a lime Popsicle. The chemo really influences the taste buds, so even though this was a lime Popsicle, there really wasn't much flavor to it; it just felt really good to be able to chew something again.

During this stay I started getting my growth hormone shots. I took these to boost the production of my stem cells so I could harvest them and then auto transplant them after round three of chemo. I had never given myself shots before and wasn't sure I could do it, but after one of the nurses, Gary, showed me how to do it, it wasn't so bad. The needles are very small and sharp, and if I pinched my skin while injecting the shot, I didn't feel any pain at all.

Dr. Hernandez came by to say that I would have to continue taking vanco for about two more weeks and that I would have to get about ten growth hormone shots. He said I wasn't going home for at least two more days; confirming that I would celebrate my 53rd birthday in Roswell. Good news though, my vitamin K shots are now in pill form.

Tuesday, January 21, 2003

Happy Birthday to Me!

I ate breakfast at about 8:30 a.m. I'm feeling pretty good today, but a little bummed that I might have to spend my birthday in Roswell. I am on what is commonly called the "Roswell Diet". At the end of my second round of chemo I have lost a total of forty pounds. None of my clothes fit and I am looking forward to getting some new pants and shirts. This is the lowest I have been in many years and it feels strange, but good.

Around lunch time the doctor came in and said if I felt like it, I could go home. I thought he was kidding – he didn't smile or anything. But sure enough, he meant it, so I got to spend half of my birthday at home. My birthday supper was a couple of pierogies and half a pork chop. I never had a better birthday dinner.

Friday, January 24, 2003

I gave myself my last dose of vanco yesterday. Now I could sleep through the night without worrying about getting up to do an infusion. I had a visit at Roswell yesterday for blood, platelets and regular fluids. It was just another typical, five-hour visit to the clinic. I have my next appointment for 9:30 a.m. Sunday. The visiting nurse is supposed to pay a visit today. Before she got there, I was able to sneak in a quick, hot shower. What a great feeling.

When I got out of the shower, the house seemed cold. I checked the furnace and it wasn't functioning. I managed to coerce the furnace repair guy to come to the house by saying I was home alone, I was very ill and needed the heat. He got there about an hour later and it cost over $200.00 to fix. At least it's warm again. I began wondering if another set of "three" was about to occur.

I no sooner got settled than the visiting nurse stopped by to check up on me and answer any questions I had. I must say that the visiting nurses (usually the same one, Jan) were fantastic. Very friendly and they took their time to make sure I understood everything and that I didn't need anything. The guys from Upstate Pharmacy supplied most of my drugs and they were also amazing. I could call and say I needed a refill or some new drug, and they were at the house within forty-five minutes, even in the worst weather.

Sunday, January 26, 2003

I spent another five hours in the infusion clinic today. I received fluids, blood and platelets. The platelets were actually donated to me from one of my co-workers at Buffalo State College – Julie Dougherty.

I can't stress enough how important it is for people to donate blood and platelets. It's a painless process that can save many lives.

I was still getting my growth hormone shots, but it turned out that Carla was better at giving me the shots than I was giving them to myself. I guess I was just being a "big baby".

I had a severe case of "cabin fever" today. These were the times that were hard to handle, and I experienced these feelings after the first round of chemo too, but this time they seemed worse. I was feeling very good, and almost good enough to go back to work. But of course, I had no immune system and the smallest cold could have been deadly for me. Besides, even though I felt good, the least little exertion tired me out. So, I was stuck in the house, totally bored.

HARVESTING STEM CELLS
Tuesday, January 28, 2003

I had my stem cells harvested today. If Keith from the pheresis clinic hadn't called, I would have been in big trouble. I was supposed to be paying attention to my white count and when it got over 10,000 I was supposed to be in the pheresis clinic so they could be harvested and frozen. If I missed that and the counts got too high, I would be back to square one and in serious shape with my health. As it was, when I got there for them to harvest my cells, my count was over 11,000. I made it just under the wire.

Pheresis is a procedure in which the blood is filtered, separated, and a portion retained, with the remainder being returned to the patient. The process was very simple. They hooked up my port to a couple of lines. One took my blood out and into a machine where it was divided into red cells, platelets, and stem cells. They kept the platelets and stem cells and infused the red cells back into me using the other port. The whole process took about three hours and was painless. I got to lie on the bed, watch TV, and eat whatever I wanted.

The rest of the month was fairly quiet. I called Barbara Anderson, from the bone marrow transplant clinic, to find out what was on the schedule. She said I would have to come back to Roswell for a dental check up, a MUG-A scan, chest x-ray, pulmonary function test and arterial gases tests. Sounded like fun; I had already had everything except the arterial gases test, so I wasn't worried. And going to the dentist shouldn't be a big deal. Before Barbara hung up she said, "By the way, you have to have a bone marrow biopsy too."

While I was at the clinic I was given a gallon jug and told to fill it up. Over the next twenty-four hours, whenever I had to urinate, I had to use my jug. When it was full, Carla drove me in so I could drop it off at the hematology clinic. When I got there, they looked at me like, "What are we supposed to do with this?" After I explained who I was and that the doctor told me to drop it off, they accepted it, but I never found out what they did with it.

Friday, January 31, 2003

The second of the "three" occurred today. Brett and Collett came to visit and we learned that Brett's mom was in the hospital with a blood clot on her brain. The doctors said it didn't look good for her. Even though Brett and Collett were busy with work and school, they were strong and brave during this time. I don't know if I could have handled this as well as they did when I was their age.

Wednesday, February 5, 2003

February was moving along fairly quietly, no major issues or burps. I was feeling pretty good and even ventured out of the house for a couple of hours. I had to wear a mask over my mouth and nose so I wouldn't inhale any germs. It seemed a little weird going places with it on, but most people just ignored it.

Several people came to the house to visit and brought food. I didn't want to tell them that I had to be careful about how my food was prepared, and probably couldn't eat any of what they brought me. One friend brought me her "famous" tuna noodle casserole. I was really tempted to eat some of it until I discovered that she simply added a can of tuna fish to Kraft macaroni and cheese and baked it for half an hour. I didn't eat any of it.

Collett had her college computer home, so for a change of routine, I started cleaning it up, removing old files and viruses, etc. It seemed to take a lot longer than I thought it would and even though I was mostly just sitting, watching the machine do its thing, I was very tired when I was done.

About this time I started having bad dreams whenever I went to sleep. These dreams mostly consisted of my losing my job or having our house foreclosed. I think part of it was also worrying about round three of chemo; another part of it was just the fact that I had so many strange chemicals coursing through my body. The doctor said it could take as much as a year for the residual chemicals to be completely flushed from my system. I think I was also worrying about using up all my sick days and vacation time. I was getting pretty low and had a long way to go. I was fortunate that I had accumulated 200 sick days and over thirty vacation days. I managed to get through the whole process without ever leaving the state payroll system. I know many people are not that fortunate.

Friday, February 7, 2003

Today was better than most. I have had a lot of low days. I am totally frustrated and have a sense of being out of control. I feel good and want to do things, but just walking up a flight of stairs tires me out. I get to the top and have forgotten why I was there, so I just laid down on the bed and took an hour-long "nap". Carla tells me that the chemo and leukemia have changed me mentally and physically, and that I should learn to chill out. She says I need to be more patient and learn to be flexible, and go with the flow, so to speak. I don't think that will ever happen with me. My personality is stronger than the drugs, and I'm just too stubborn to change.

Everyone tells me how brave and strong I am. I try to be gracious and say, "Thank you", but the will to live is stronger in me than I thought. I looked at it as if I had only two choices. I could do one of two things: give in and let the leukemia win or fight like hell and say this isn't the way I planned to die. And to my surprise, it really didn't have anything to do with "all those things I haven't done yet", or "I want to live to see my grand kids". I just didn't feel like giving in. I had had all of the common childhood illnesses -- chicken pox, measles, mumps, and I had my tonsils and adenoids removed when I was two years old. I was just going to prove that I could beat this thing.

I think having Carla and Collett behind me giving me all their support and always being positive certainly helped. If I was alone, I don't know if I would have survived.

Collett was in her second year of college at SUNY Geneseo and I think I was putting on a "brave" front so she wouldn't worry so much that it impacted her studies. At the time, her boyfriend, Brett, was with her at school and he was able to give her some support. But his mother was ill, too, and we didn't know her fate from day to day.

Saturday, February 8, 2003

Brett's mother had surgery to remove the blood clot on her brain. She was in a hospital in Buffalo and Brett was staying with us so he wouldn't have to commute between Buffalo and Rochester. He was going through a tough time, and

I think he and Collett were consoling each other, and giving each other moral support to get through all of this mess.

Tuesday, February 11, 2003

Today was another one of those frustrating days. I was feeling really good and wanted to go back to work; I knew I couldn't. I was feeling a little antsy today and wanted to do something besides sit around the house. But still, the least little exertion tired me out. I still couldn't get warm, no matter how many clothes I wore.

TEST DAY
Wednesday, February 12, 2003

Today's the day. I have tests at Roswell scheduled from 8:30 a.m. through late afternoon.

The first appointment was with the dentist. I was told that dental hygiene is very important because if I have cavities or other oral issues, the bacteria and germs that grow could affect my whole body. This is because the chemo stripped my system of its immune system and the tiniest germ could make me very sick.

The next test was the MUG-A, where radioactive dye is injected into me; after that my heart is photographed with a special type of x-ray machine. Over 100 images of my heart are taken in about a half hour. This is to see what effects the chemo had had on my heart, and to make sure it's still functioning properly.

From there, I went to the Pulmonary Functions Lab, where I had my arterial gases tested. This is a test to see how much oxygen, CO_2, and other gases my blood is holding and processing. From the name of the test, it should be obvious that blood has to be taken from an artery. The only artery that is close enough to the surface to do this test is located in the wrist. As my luck would have it, it took the technician two tries to find a suitable artery. The whole process takes only five minutes or so, but because my platelet count was so low, it took almost 10 minutes to stop the bleeding.

I had a test to see how well my lungs were functioning. I was locked into a glass box, and I had to breathe through a small tube. I guess they were measuring how much air I could inhale and exhale. Now I know how a pilot feels when he or she is in the cockpit of an airplane. There was no airflow in the box, and it got very warm, very quickly. I was sweating when I was done with the tests.

I also had an EKG and chest x-rays done; a urine analysis; and eight vials of blood were drawn.

To finish off the day in great style, I had one more bone marrow biopsy! This one also took two attempts. For some reason, Dr. Wetzler couldn't get through my bone and into the marrow. What should have been about a half hour took almost a full hour to get done. Part of the problem was my stubbornness in refusing to use "conscious sedation". By the time I got home, I was tired and sore. My "counts" are looking good and right now I'm scheduled to return on February 24th for the third round of chemo and the stem cell transplant.

Valentine's Day
Friday, February 14, 2003

A visiting nurse from Univera stopped by to check up on me today. I was always amazed at how friendly, professional and caring the staff members seemed to be during any visit. All of my vital signs were good, and I was feeling good. After answering all of my questions, she left.

Carla surprised me today with a card, marzipan and some chocolate. This is the first time in our thirty-two years of marriage that I didn't get Carla a Valentine's card or candy. I was not allowed to drive, or basically, leave the house alone.

In about six more weeks, I would know if I achieved remission or not. When I am declared "infusion-independent", the Hickman catheter would be removed and I could start getting back to normal.

Saturday, February 15, 2003

Collett called today to say that Brett's mom had passed. I'm not sure if he even had a chance to say good-bye. He and his mom were pretty close and he was trying to help Collett cope with my illness at the same time. I think it was pretty rough on him, but he never talked about it. I couldn't do much to support Collett or Brett. I felt bad for both of them because I wasn't able to attend the funeral.

Sunday, February 16, 2003

I called this our "slug" day. I didn't know it at the time, but today started a trend that lasts even to today. Neither Carla nor I even got out of pajamas, didn't take a shower, and pretty much dozed the day away. Sunday's are now our lazy days and we make an effort to not schedule anything to do.

The days have been passing quietly. The weather has been lousy, so I had no desire to go outside for anything. The high spots of my day were going out for the mail, and later going back out to get the newspaper, after which it took an hour to warm up. I was drinking a lot of tea now to help me get warm and I snuck in some honey from time to time.

I'm looking forward to getting the third round of chemo done and over with. I am optimistically planning to return to work, at least part time; by mid-May 2003 (this turned out to be very optimistic on my part).

THE DENTIST APPOINTMENT
Wednesday, February 19, 2003

Roswell is very much self-contained. Any service you need could be provided by some department somewhere in the hospital. I assumed this was because they knew how to deal with cancer patients in various states of treatment and/or remission and it was easier just to keep all the records in one place. The only catch seems to be that the different departments don't talk to each other.

Because I had a port, I was supposed to get antibiotics before seeing the dentist. I was in the chair, ready to go, when the dentist or hygienist ask me how I was doing. I said, "Fine, I am glad to have the port so I don't get stuck so many times." Well, she got all excited, said, "No one told me about your port! You need medication before I can continue."

So, I got a shot of penicillin and was told to come back in an hour, after the drugs had a chance to get through my system. I was having trouble with the lines anyway; the red line was slow infusing. So I stopped by the pain clinic to have it checked out, and to kill some time. Well, I needed something called "TPA", which of course was frozen and would have to thaw before it could be infused into my port's red line. I went out to the little café in the lobby and had a cup of coffee and a bagel while I was waiting for the "TPA" to thaw.

I finally got the TPA and the line was working better. I went back up to the dentist. Now I was 40 minutes "late" for my appointment and I had to wait for all the patients who were on time.

All the normal procedures were done; x-rays – including a 180-degree, panoramic view, scraping some plaque off my teeth, digging to see if they could find any cavities, and so on. Finally, it was time to clean my teeth. The dentist used this spray device that shot out some powder similar to baking soda – a real fine powdery spray. It wasn't so bad at first, but after about five minutes I began to know how a building feels when it gets sand blasted.

My thirty-minute visit that started at 1:00 p.m. was now done at 3:00 p.m. No visit to Roswell is ever less than two hours.

I was due in the Pain Clinic for my weekly check up, and I thought I was going to be late because of the dentist. Dr. Wetzler wanted to pull my line because it wasn't working properly. After some poking and prodding by one of the nurses, it was determined that the blue line was okay and the red line would infuse, but not draw. So, the line was left in.

Thursday, February 20, 2003

I actually managed to get to "work" today for a few minutes. If the doctor knew, he would have shot me. Nothing there really changed much from the time I left. I visited a few offices and it was fun. I had no hair, facial or otherwise, and was wearing a baseball cap the people in the library had given me. I would sit somewhere and wait for someone I knew to walk by. I'd say something like, "Well, don't even say hi." The person would stop a few steps later, turn around and glare at me, like, "Why are you bothering me?" Then the light came on, they would smile and come back to talk to me. I got a lot of hugs this way.

I think being able to get out of the house and do normal things was a big boost. I felt a little depressed and gloomy. I probably wasn't supposed to drive, but I just had to get out of the house. The concern was that since I have a very low platelet count, if I were to get into an accident I could bleed to death internally.

It's not like things at work needed attending to. My two graduate students, Debbie and Sara, were pretty much running the place. They even implemented some procedures I had been meaning to put in place to help with scheduling and training. I am glad they were there to cover for me. When I look back, it almost seems like this was supposed to happen. I was at a time in my life where I had no direction and needed something to get me back on track.

When I got home I was tired and had to lie down. Four more days of freedom before I headed back to Roswell for round three.

ROUND THREE BEGINS
Monday, February 24, 2003

Carla drove me to Roswell today, and I checked in for round three at about 9:00 a.m. I was able to be on five-west again. I think this helped, too, because I knew all the nurses and support staff, so it almost seemed like coming home. By now we are expert at the process of checking in, getting set up in my room, changing clothes and all of that.

For this round of chemo I will be taking Busulfan (intended for intravenous administration. It is supplied as a clear, colorless, sterile, solution) and Etoposide VP-16 (reduce the production of white blood cells by the bone marrow).

In the first two rounds of chemo I suffered from mucositis, which made it very difficult to eat, chew and swallow.

Mucositis is the inflammation of your mucous membranes, which are tissues that line your digestive system – all the way from your mouth, esophagus, stomach, intestines, and rectum to your anus. Mucositis is caused when chemotherapy attacks and kills the rapidly dividing cells in your mucous membranes. So you have trouble brushing your teeth.

Dr. Sullivan, one of the dentists at Roswell, stopped by for me to sign some papers. I had volunteered for a new dental protocol and I was going to be the guinea pig to test a new mouthwash for patients with mucositis. The stuff tasted terrible, but it did ease some of the pain I was having in my mouth.

On top of this, the chemo aggravated my hemorrhoids. Nothing the doctors or nurses tried helped with this pain. There was one humorous note to this however. During an especially bad bout of pain, nurse Lucia (who specialized in this kind of thing) stopped by to see if she could help. She refers to herself as the "Butt Queen". She had me turn my butt towards the window and opened the blinds so she could get more light. After I got situated she had to leave the room to get some cream, and told me, "Don't move." Now, I'm on the fifth floor of Roswell Park Cancer Institute, thinking, "Who in the world is going to see my naked butt hanging out there?" Well, out of nowhere, down drops the window washer! I am sure he was as surprised as I was when he stopped to clean my windows. He didn't hang around long, you can be sure of that. This incident caused a change in hospital policy. From that point on, any maintenance to the outside of the building had to be announced in writing, and various department heads had to sign off saying they were aware of the maintenance and that no patients would be exposed to such a thing again. Several of the nurses "cracked" up over this and I was the "butt" of jokes for a few days.

Kim Sweeney also stopped by to give me the "game plan" for round three of chemo. Today is day-8. Negative numbers are used because it's a way of counting down to transplant day. So, eight days from today I would receive my auto transplant.

Dr. Slack stopped by to tell me I had elevated liver counts. He said at this point he couldn't determine what was causing the elevation. He said he would keep an eye on the counts. He was concerned that my liver counts could interfere with my transplant. (Shortly after his visit we found out why my liver counts were elevated – Collett had been exposed to mononucleosis before one of her visits to see me.)

Dr. Slack also said that most people returned to work in three to six months. This was mostly due to the fact that after having chemo, I would tire easily and my immune system would still be too weak to protect me from the germs at work. This meant that I would not be able to go back to work until July at the earliest and October at the latest. But he did say that if I remained leukemia free for three years, I would be considered cured. (Dr. Wetzler called it long term remission.)

I was beginning to wonder if all of this time, pain, grief, and depression would be worth it. I was wondering if I had wasted the last four months of my life and if all of the medical procedures would really extend my life. There were days when, honestly, I really didn't care either way. The doctors and nurses had said that during this process there would be good days, bad days, and really bad days.

Tuesday, February 25, 2003

According to Gary, one of the nurses in the ward, I am taking Busulfan in place of getting radiation treatments. The Busulfan might cause seizures, so I am taking Dilantin to prevent the seizures. I am taking something called a loaded dose of the Busulfan, but I'm not sure what that means. After this initial dose, I will start getting the medication every eight hours – over the next four days I will get sixteen doses of the Busulfan.

Sleep in a hospital always seems to be an issue. If the nurses wanting to take vitals do not awaken me, the aides come in to leave clean linens or to clean my bathroom. The side effects of the drugs also make it hard to sleep or even to relax. Some of the drugs cause hallucinations or nightmares. By looking at the entries in my journal I can always tell when my drugs have changed; either a different dosage or a new drug added. It's funny now to look back at my journal to try to figure out what in the world I was trying to say. Some pages look like a two-year old wrote them.

While I was in the hospital, I kept a small basket filled with chocolate, mini candy bars and hard candy on the shelf in my room. I didn't eat much of it, but every time someone came into my room for something, I made sure they left with at least one piece of candy. After a while I had people coming in just for the candy, but that was okay.

Tuesday, February 26, 2003

The chemo has started. "Barney" is loaded up with the chemo drugs and fluids. There is no effect yet, but the effects usually are not felt until about fourteen days after the drugs have been infused.

Both of my ports are in use with the chemicals for the chemo. I need two injections of Dilantin, and soon I will be getting growth hormone shots. To alleviate the need to find different places to stick me, a mini-port was inserted into my left arm. The doctors and nurses can reuse this port for four or five days, then a new one has to be inserted. It sure beats getting stuck eight or nine times a day.

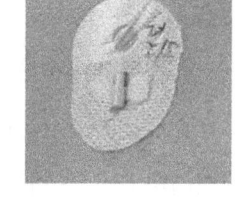

Figure 6 Mini-port

Thursday, February 27, 2003

Today I had my dressings changed, but because I had my medical pump attached, I couldn't take a shower. I am learning to appreciate the little things in life again -- things I took for granted for so many years – a hot shower, clean clothes, clean bed linens, and the freedom to move around as I wanted.

We found out today that Carla's mom, Ruby Mae, is in the hospital with pancreatitis. I hope she is doing well and gets to go home soon. Carla has too much to worry about now -- Collett, her work, the house, herself, and me. I wish she would go home to Oneida and visit. I don't know why she doesn't go. I am in good hands here and I don't think anything will happen right away.

According to the system used here, I am at Day-6. In just six more days I get my transplant and then maybe home. It's only been three days, but already it seems like a lot longer.

It's interesting to note what things seem to stick in my mind while waiting for my transplant. The news on TV said that Mr. Rogers died today. He was 75 years old. I was wondering if I would make it to 75. One patient died while I was here in round three. The nurses came around and closed all the doors so we wouldn't see the body being taken out. It was a little depressing to think that some people come here and never get to go home.

I don't know if it's because of the side effects of the drugs or if it's because Roswell is just always cold, but Carla notices that I am shaking a lot. I know it's not from drinking coffee because I gave that up during round two. Coffee just started tasting bad and I couldn't stomach it. Even the tea started tasting bad.

THE TRANSPLANT
Sunday, March 1, 2003

Today is Day-3 and I got my last round of chemotherapy (Etoposide VP-16). It took four hours to infuse and one of the nurses had to take my vitals every half hour to make sure I am doing okay and not having any major side effects.

I did get nauseous and vomited a little. I immediately was reprimanded for vomiting. Chemo makes everything very sensitive; my skin was very thin and cut easily, my platelet count was non-existent, so any tears or cuts could cause me to bleed excessively. The nurses were afraid that if I vomited I might tear my esophagus and that would lead to major bleeding and complications. They put enough fear into me so that anytime I started to feel ill again, I immediately called them for anti-nausea medication.

The doctor told me that the third round of chemo would be the worst. It had pretty much ravaged my body with all the different chemicals. When I looked back at my journal I could definitely tell when the effects of the chemo hit me. My journal looks like I was writing with a blunt, black crayon instead of a pen.

Later, around 11:00 a.m., I tried to sleep, but was having hallucinations. I swore that Carla was standing next to my bed talking to me and that she had brought me some candy and a book. Some sound startled me awake, and I realized that I was alone in my room.

One of the maintenance crew, William, took a liking to me. He arranged his cleaning schedule so he would do my room last. He and I chatted quite a bit on a variety of topics, but mostly about the lottery. He was always telling me what numbers were hot and which ones were cold. He even bought me a scratch-off ticket once and I won five dollars. He said I could keep it, but I asked him to buy more tickets with it. I never won again.

Sunday, March 2, 2003

After the chemo and before the transplant, the body is supposed to "rest". So, I was resting. Resting basically means no chemo or unnecessary drugs. I was still connected to "Barney" to be sure I was getting enough fluids.

Dr. Hernandez stopped by to let me know my white cell count was very high. This was of concern because a high white cell count is what put me here in the first place. The doctor said my high white count was probably due to all the meds I was on. He ordered a chest X-ray and a couple of other tests, just to be on the safe side.

Monday, March 3, 2003

Tomorrow I start my stem cell transplant. Collett had visited as often as she could, but between school and work, it was hard to get back to Buffalo. When I did see her, she seemed to always be tired and run down. I was concerned that she was working too hard and not getting enough sleep. Collett came in to visit today and hit us with some interesting news. She had finally gone to see a doctor and she was told that she had mononucleosis. Dr. Wetzler was very upset and concerned about my well-being. I had absolutely no immune system, but I had to go through with the transplant. If I had contracted mono that could possibly influence the outcome of the transplant. The doctor immediately started a course of medication to protect my liver and (hopefully), avoid any complications. Collett was banned from the hospital and couldn't come back to visit for the rest of the time I was in Roswell. She wasn't even allowed to come into the waiting room.

Because of this, I was also considered infectious. They couldn't throw me out of the hospital, but did the next best thing. I could not leave my room unless I was wearing a mask, a gown and rubber gloves. Anyone who came into my room had to wear a mask and had to sanitize their hands before entering and after leaving. Needless to say, I did not leave my room much after that.

Tuesday, March 4, 2003

Today's the day. It's 11:00 a.m., and the transfusion has started. Dr. Wetzler said that I could have visitors during the transfusion/transplant and that different people experienced different smells during the transfusion. Carla said she smelled creamed corn. I didn't smell anything, but I had a funny taste in my mouth.

I had two bags of stems cells to infuse, so the whole process took about an hour. I was given Benadryl, so I slept through most of the process. Barbara Anderson, the transplant coordinator, stayed in my room through the whole process, explaining what was going on. It's a simple process, but can have a major impact on the person getting the stem cells.

Because of my exposure to mono, there were concerns about hepatitis B & C. I could have gotten hepatitis C because of the tattoo I had gotten a couple of years earlier and B from the mono. My liver enzymes were down, but still elevated above normal. So, the doctors took a "wait and see" approach, and added a few more drugs to my schedule. The shaking I had experienced earlier had subsided and I was feeling pretty good.

My New Birthday

One thing that everyone at Roswell is big on is the tradition of calling the day of the transplant the patient's "New Birthday". So, forevermore, my new birthday is March 4th.

If you want every orifice and crevice in your body explored, just spend a few days in a hospital. Because of the cough I had, and because of my exposure to mono, I had to have my lungs checked for infection. James, from the infusion clinic, ran a tube through my nose and down into my lungs. He released some saline solution through the tube into my chest and then sucked it back out. Getting the tube in and out of my nose and chest was a "thrill a minute". I don't care how sick I ever get; I am <u>never</u> getting that done again.

Another side effect of getting chemo is depression. It hits people at different times during or after a transplant. My first bout came later in the day of my transplant. When I knew I was alone and would not have anyone dropping in on me, I would sit in the chair in my room and cry. Usually not long, five or ten minutes, and then I would pull myself together and carry on as the big, brave, macho person I was trying to be. This depression would lead to my being put on Paxil for a short time. Getting on and off Paxil was almost worse than the depression itself. (The depression returned five years later.) The depression seemed to come in bouts. Some days were worse than others.

During most of my treatments I tried to keep a "normal" schedule. I somehow knew I was going to beat this and I wanted to be ready to go back to work. I would force myself to get up and out of bed by 8:30 a.m. each day (sometimes the nurses helped with this, although unwittingly); I would take a cat bath, brush my teeth and write in my journal until breakfast came. I would eat breakfast, watch some TV and write in my journal again until lunch. Usually after lunch the physical therapist would come around and we would toss a medicine ball around for a while; I would do some stretching exercises; and lift small weights. If nothing else, it helped break up the day and give me something to look forward to. I knew a lot of patients would get out of bed only long enough for the aides to change the sheets and clean their rooms. I know attitude had a lot to do with me getting better.

One more side effect was the taste of food. This is different for everyone and for me everything tasted sweet. I couldn't eat potato chips (probably a good thing) because they tasted like they were coated with sugar instead of salt. Candy of any sort tasted doubly sweet and I stopped eating that too.

At this point, I have lost over fifty pounds. My only regret is that I didn't keep it off.

Monday, March 5, 2003

It's the first full day after my transplant. If I wasn't so depressed, I'd feel pretty good, good enough to go home. The dietician was just here and I planned next week's meals. Even this is getting monotonous; the food doesn't even sound good any more.

I can't eat because I can't swallow; I can't breathe because my nose is plugged; I feel so tired. I'm depressed and it's too easy to let the depression take over. I want to be "healed" and get back to my normal routine. The doctor put me on Entac™ for my nasal congestion, but this elevated my blood pressure so I was switched to Flonase™, which seemed to work just as well, but didn't affect my blood pressure. (I'm still taking it.)

Dr. Wetzler stopped by to say my liver enzymes were going down, but there was a small up-blip that concerned him. He says I need to stay at least two more weeks to be sure everything is okay. I might make it home by the end of March. Talk about being depressed!

I was warned that the third round of chemo would be the worst. I have been trying hard to stay upbeat, but this round is finally making me ask, "Why me?" "What did I do to deserve this?"

When I came in for my first round of chemo, I looked at the doctors and nurses as special. I thought they were above average people in many ways. This round of chemo has made me see them as just regular people with their own problems, trying to do the best they can for the people for whom they are caring for. But I still see them as heroes, because they do work hard. They seem to put aside their personal concerns and concentrate on the needs of the patients.

I was shocked to learn that most of the nurses would take their breaks outside so they could smoke. They make an effort to cover the cigarette smell, but sometimes it's easy to smell it on their breaths and clothes.

Thursday, March 6, 2003

It is 8:00 a.m. and I am trying to maintain my routine of writing for a while as I waited for breakfast to arrive. I was feeling good, but it was still early in the day -- a lot of things could change. I haven't had a shower since February 23rd and the cat baths just weren't cutting it anymore.

I've been here only eleven days for this round of chemo, but it seems like an eternity. Dr. Wetzler says that I should be home by the end of March – 23 more days. I will definitely be insane by then. I think I was starting to get the feeling of being isolated from the world. I couldn't do what I wanted to, when I wanted to; I missed my family and I just felt like I was out of the loop, as they say.

There was a Chevy commercial on TV about going to a place that nobody knows. I got a copy of the full poem and it goes like this:

Nobody Knows It but Me[5]

There's a place I travel
when I want to roam,
and nobody knows it but me.
The roads don't go there
and signs stay home,
and nobody knows it but me.
It's far, far away and way, way afar.
it's over the moon and the sea.
And wherever you're going
that's wherever you are.
And nobody knows it but me.

By Patrick O'Leary © General Motors 2002

---

[5] With permission of the author

Whenever I get truly depressed I read this poem and pretend I am in this place, far, far away. It helps for a few minutes and it takes away all the pain and depression I feel.

One thing about this hospital is that it was run on a very regular schedule. Except for weekends I could expect someone to come into my room around 6:30 a.m. and drop off clean linens; at 8:00 a.m. the cleaning crew came in to empty waste baskets, refill toilet paper, etc. and they were not quiet as they went about their chores; around 9:00 a.m., breakfast is delivered and the day started.

Dr. Wetzler came back to say my liver enzymes are elevated and that I might be getting an IVIG infusion – this is Immunoglobulin – because of my exposure to some form of mono.

Because of the risk to the other patients on the ward, I was placed in real isolation. Anyone coming into my room had to wear a mask, gown and gloves so they would not carry the mono infection out of my room. Whenever I left the room I had to wear a mask, gloves, and a gown to help prevent the spread of the mono. It became a very depressing time for me and I stopped leaving my room unless one of the nurses nagged me long enough to get up and get some exercise. The "threat" of not being able to go home was a very effective motivator.

Friday, March 7, 2003

I am practicing for my time in a nursing home. Like a good patient, I am newly bathed, teeth brushed, and sitting in the chair in my room waiting for breakfast, a visit from doctor, and any odd visitor who might show up.

Dr. Wetzler stopped by for a few minutes to see how I was doing, and to tell me that I wouldn't need the IVIG shots after all. That was good news! All I needed was one more drug added to the list.

Saturday, March 8, 2003

Darlene, one of the aides in the ward, weighed me today. Technology is really great. My bed had a built-in scale so I didn't even have to get out of bed to be weighed. Today I weighed 113KG or about 249 pounds. This was the first time I had been less than 250 pounds for a very long time. I had lost approximately fifty pounds since the beginning of this trip. The "Roswell Diet" works very well.

Sunday, March 9, 2003

Another weekend in this place and I started it off right. Rick, the nurse, and Gail, the aide, stopped by to see me and to "steal" some of my candy. I don't know what did it, but I started crying and just could not stop. I've never felt like a bigger baby in my life. I didn't know if I was breaking down and going crazy, or if I was just physically exhausted from the schedule of drugs and the "after effects" of the chemo. I felt so hopeless and drained that I began sleeping away most of the days.

Tuesday, March 11, 2003

The day started with me watching TV as usual. A commercial came on about some local school (I think it was the Hunting Learning Center); the main character came into the kitchen and her mom asked her how she did on her final project. The young girl smiled and said she received an A on her paper. I started bawling like a little baby. To this day I don't know why. It took a while before I could stop.

Later in the day Dr. Wetzler and a group of medical students stopped by to check up on me. They found me curled up in bed in a fetal position crying my eyes out. I just couldn't stop. I kept apologizing for my behavior – that macho thing, where men don't cry, was cropping up again.

He immediately ordered a diet of clear liquids and had a morphine pump attached to "Barney". I could control the dosages by pressing a button. Dr. Wetzler explained that depression was sometimes a side effect of the chemo and that after three rounds of the stuff, my mind and body had been through quite a lot. An appointment was made for me to talk to a counselor to discuss my issues. My conversations resulted in me being prescribed Paxil.

I don't know if was the chemo, the morphine, or my body just being exhausted from being abused by all these drugs, but sleeping became a real problem. When I did sleep I had nightmares. I would wake up at odd hours of the night and hallucinate, thinking I was home or out in a field some place. The bed also seemed to be harder this time and less comfortable.

Eating has become a problem again. Every time I tried to eat, I got nauseous. I had to have a Fenergan patch (A phenothiazine derivative with histamine H1-blocking, antimuscarinic, and sedative properties. It is used as an antiallergic, in pruritus, for motion sickness and sedation) put on my shoulder.

I had developed an infection in my nose, so I was also getting Albuterol (a bronchodilator used in treating asthma and other conditions with reversible airway obstruction) treatments. This is in the form of an inhaler. I had to breathe in this vapor a couple of times a day to help clear up my nasal/sinus infection.

My diet has changed again. I was now on a soft, low, microbial diet. This meant I got to eat things like bananas and eggs. But it was hard to chew because of the mucusitis. I feel like Goldilocks; I couldn't eat anything that is too hot or too cold, it had to be "just right" (something that remains to this day). My energy levels are low and I am losing any ambition to do anything. This is obvious by looking at the entries in my journal – they are getting very terse and days go by without any entries.

GOING HOME AT LAST
Sunday, March 16, 2003

I got discharged today and was able to make it home. I felt like I was hit with a Mac Truck, but just the thought of leaving the hospital and getting back to my own bed and environment was enough to keep me moving. The risk of fever and infection was still very high, so I have to keep an eye on my temperature. We bought a new thermometer that took my temperature via my ear, just like the ones in the hospital.

Monday, March 17, 2003
Saint Patrick's Day

Even though I was discharged yesterday, today is the first full day at home and I used this date to mark my anniversary of leaving Roswell Park Cancer Institute.

I guess I was too used to the hospital routine. I had a hard time sleeping and I woke up about every four hours. I was also having nightmares and I know I kept Carla awake.

Carla stayed home with me for most of the day, but she needed to have her corned beef and cabbage for Saint Paddy's day. Just the thought of it made me nauseous.

Tuesday, March 18, 2003

Out of the hospital one day, and I already have to go back for a bone marrow biopsy. This time I get to go to 5-North, the bone marrow transplant clinic. I am making my own new blood and platelets, although both are still a little low.

I have been taken off almost all my meds. Only Acyclovar, Protonix, and Regalan are left. My hemorrhoids are still acting up, still aggravated by the chemo that my body is trying to get rid of.

At this point I am visiting Roswell every three or four days. Most of the visits are just for checkups, but sometimes I have to go the infusion clinic for fluids and blood work.

Wednesday, March 19, 2003

I think this is Day+15, but I've lost count. The sores in my mouth have cleared up and I was able to eat a bowl of cereal for breakfast. This is progress.

Sharon, a Univera visiting nurse, stopped by today to check up on me. She gave me a clean bill of health; my blood pressure was good and my lungs were clear.

It has been almost five months since this adventure started. Looking back now, the time seems to have gone by quickly. I am looking forward to being able to ride my bicycle and just being outdoors again.

Thursday, March 20, 2003

I had another visit to the bone marrow transplant clinic today. Pam, the nurse practitioner, says everything is going as expected. I was taken off most of my medications -- just acyclovir, protonix (decreases the amount of acid produced in the stomach), and regalan (Regalan increases the contractions of the stomach and small intestine, helping the passage of food) are left. My red blood count and platelet counts continue to increase – that was good news. I would be making several more visits to the clinic.

Monday, March 24, 2003

I visited the bone marrow transplant clinic again, for a routine checkup. There were concerns about how chemo affects the brain and memory. So, I volunteered for a study with some psychologists to examine the effects of chemo on the brain. I didn't tell them my memory was messed up before I started chemo.

Wednesday, March 26, 2003

My medical port was removed today. It took about twenty minutes to get the device out because there seemed to be some issues with it. And of course, what would a visit to Roswell be without another bone marrow biopsy?

The good feelings were quickly dampened when we got home from Roswell. Carla's brother had called to say her mom, Ruby Mae Collett, had passed away in her sleep that day. She was supposed to go play bingo with one of her friends, but said she needed a little nap. Her friend came to pick up to go to bingo, but could not wake her up. Hopefully, Ruby passed peacefully and didn't suffer – she was 76 years old. (This was the third item in the new group of "three".)

We took a trip to Oneida to make arrangements for Carla's mom to be buried. I couldn't have felt worse; it was like

I had been run over by a horse and carriage and then backed over by a big truck. But I had to be there to attempt to support Carla.

Sunday, March 30, 2003

Because of the weather and the ground being so hard, Ruby could not be buried until the end of March. Carla, Collett and I made it to Oneida for her mother's funeral. It was a nice day and a sad day at the same time. It was nice to have everyone together (it had been a long time since we had been home) and sad of course, because of the occasion for us getting together. It's been a tough year. I don't know how Carla handled all of this. In many ways, she is much stronger than I am.

Tuesday, April 15, 2003

It's been about a month now since I was discharged. My life is getting back to normal. I was still making weekly visits to Roswell for blood work and infusion when I needed them. Other than my hemorrhoids bothering me, I felt pretty good. I was eating a little better than before, but I was still not eating fresh fruit or vegetables; it takes too much time to prepare them, and Carla has to do all the work.

Friday, April 25, 2003

Today started with another appointment at Roswell. We arrived a little early to get the blood work done and to have lunch before I see the doctor. Carla was with me today and we meet with Laura, the physician's assistant. My platelet count was okay, but not where it was expected to be. Laura thinks my mono has come back, so I am taken back into the infusion clinic and given an Intravenous immunoglobulin treatment (IVIG). We had not expected this, and spent the rest of the day receiving IVs. This was the first of five infusions, so I would have to come back every day for the next five days; spending at least two hours at Roswell for each infusion. Because my catheter had been removed, I had to deal with being injected. I forgot how much those injections hurt. I did learn, however, that doctors and nurses like to start "low" when doing injections. That is, they start in the hand. If they can't get a good vein there, they move up to the arm, and then further up until they get a good vein. This is done because if they start "high" and have to move down to get a good vein, the vein could leak and the drugs would not be infused properly.

Today I was put back on acyclovir and the anti-depressant Paxil. If my counts didn't come back up, I wouldn't have to get a bone marrow biopsy on Monday.

Today's visit to Roswell started at noon and we left at 6:00 p.m. Any support person, family, and friends are impacted by leukemia and its treatment as much as the patient. I am very grateful that Carla was always so patient and attentive. She kept me in check because I am not (and have never been) a patient person. I would have gone crazy if she wasn't there to calm me down and make me relax.

Monday, April 28, 2003

Because my numbers were moving in the wrong direction I needed to have blood work (and other tests) done to see if I had relapsed. We arrived at Roswell around 8:00 a.m. for one more bone marrow biopsy and blood work. This time I received "conscious sedation" so the biopsy went smoother. Carla says I asked the doctor what the time was about fifty times during the procedure. He just kept saying, "five minutes since the last time you asked." If I could have remembered, it would be funny. After the biopsy I had my fourth infusion of IVIG. This time wasn't so bad for me, since I slept through most of it.

One thing I learned the hard way was that it was very important for me to pay attention to what the doctors are telling me and to take extra care of myself so I didn't relapse. It was very easy to get complacent about things, thinking, I'm fine, and then doing something that sets me back in my treatment. I have decided that, at least at Roswell, the doctors really know what they are talking about and that I should be closely following their instructions.

Right now the biggest issues are the constant fatigue and feeling cold. I started feeling good, and then I would over exert myself, and paid for it by spending the next four or five hours sleeping. The feelings are like a roller coaster; I can feel really good one day and totally down in the dumps the next. I keep praying that this will even out eventually, so I can feel somewhat normal most the time.

Another issue concerned being confined at home between rounds of chemo. Even on days when I felt good, I was advised that I shouldn't be going out. I had to be concerned that I had no immune system and going out to public places put me at high risk for getting infections. And we all know how clean most restaurants and other public places are. So, I am at home, feeling fairly good and wanting to do something, but I can't. That is so frustrating and boring.

Monday, May 5, 2003

I was back in Roswell today but it was voluntary. I had an appointment with Dr. Jane Smith (honest, her real name) in the GI clinic to discuss the issue of my hemorrhoids. I guess I had them before I got sick, but I wasn't aware of it. The chemo really aggravated all of the mucus membranes in my body and even after all the chemo was done, I was still having issues.

Dr. Smith gave me some new medication to help with the swelling and the pain. It was decided that as soon as my counts were high enough I would have the surgery to have the hemorrhoids removed.

Friday, May 9, 2003

I think this is Day+66, sixty-six days since my transplant. I had to get out of the house or I would go stir crazy. I bundled myself up with sweat suit, hat, coat, gloves and mask – and headed out for a short walk. I have walked around the neighborhood before so I know some of the distances from my house. I didn't want to go so far that I couldn't get back, so I decided to walk around a short block, about ¾ of a mile. It was chilly, but the sun felt so good on my face. I must have looked pretty silly walking around the block, looking up at the sky, and wearing a mask over my nose and mouth; and of course the only masks I had were blue, so I couldn't pretend I was painting or something like that. But I didn't care; it just felt so good to be outside feeling the breeze and the warmth of the sun.

I walked at a leisurely pace, so it took me almost an hour to get around the block. It felt good to get home too. I don't think it was more than fifteen minutes after I sat down on the couch that I was fast asleep, and stayed there three hours.

One of the interesting things I noticed was that it appeared that my fingernails had three distinct "rings" or grooves going across them. It almost appeared as if my fingernails started growing after each round of chemo.

Saturday, May 10, 2003

I had noticed myself "rocking" back and forth, without the benefit of a rocking chair. I was pretty sure that this was one of the side effects the Paxil was having on me. I started walking around the house; the first floor consists of the kitchen, dining room and living room laid out in such a way that I could walk in circles, trying to burn off some of the energy, anxiety and nervousness I felt. I found out that these were known side effects, but no one bothered to warn me.

Monday, May 12, 2003

My anxiety level is at an all time high today. Carla was at work and I sat on the couch and cried for almost an hour. I was sure this was another side effect of the Paxil. I started having almost daily "fits" where I couldn't control myself. How was I supposed to get well if I felt this way all the time? I was going to try to convince the doctor to take me off the Paxil.

Saturday, May 17, 2003

It is not a good idea to quit any antidepressant all at once. I was able to get the Paxil reduced to half the dosage I was taking, but it was still a bad day today. I started off with a crying spell and then slept until about 10:30 a.m.

One good thing, I am still losing weight. At this point I weighed 224 pounds. The new clothes I had just bought were too big for me already. (Too bad I couldn't have kept the weight off.)

My days now have me starting off feeling poorly, but I forced myself to get up and attempt to do something. I always managed to eat breakfast; my taste for coffee still has not returned. Usually by mid-afternoon, I started feeling human and wanted to do things. I still couldn't get warm, and although it was May, I still wore a hat and a jacket whenever I went out.

Tuesday, May 20, 2003

I made a trip into work today. I drove myself, but I had to be careful. My platelet count was still very low and the slightest bump could have caused internal bleeding, which I guess I would not have felt. I visited with my two graduate students for about an hour and then went back home. I made a cup of tea and immediately feel asleep on the couch until Carla came home from work.

Sunday, June 1, 2003

The days are all about the same now; they are blending together. Things are slowly getting back to normal. My hair is growing back in, but it's all white; and as fine as a newborn baby's hair. Some days are better than others. I am having issues with my Paxil and hopefully will be able to stop taking it soon. My counts won't settle down and keep going up and down; the doctors can't figure out why. I feel good most of the time now, but still tire easily.

We've made several trips to Oneida. We buried Carla's mom on May 23rd. It was a nice day and about twenty friends and relatives joined us at the cemetery. Between still recovering and dealing with the funeral, both Carla and I were exhausted when we got back to Buffalo.

I visited work near the end of May to attend a library luncheon and stopped by my office to clean house a little. The days are starting out better, but I am still getting tired after only three or four hours of activity.

Friday, June 6, 2003

This is Day+95, I think; I've lost track. During my many visits to Roswell I also visited the bone marrow transplant clinic. I volunteered for another protocol where psychologists where studying the effect of chemo on memory. Today was my last "exam" and I guess I did fairly well on it. I still have a few issues with my memory, but Carla says that's just selective remembering. I jokingly say it's just old age.

Thursday, June 19, 2003

I saw Dr. Wetzler today for a routine checkup. I have to come back to Roswell about every two weeks right now. My counts were improving and he gave me permission to ride my bicycle again, but he told me to be very careful. This was good news because I planned to participate in the annual Ride for Roswell event.

Saturday, June 28, 2003

Today was the Ride for Roswell, an annual charity event that raises money for RPCI. I did the nine-mile ride in just over an hour. I had several people at work sponsor me and I think I raised about $800.00. It felt good to be outdoors riding my bicycle again. The rest of June passed quietly.

Wednesday, July 9, 2003

I needed one last operation. Today, I finally got rid of my hemorrhoids. The preparation for the surgery was disgusting and gross, but didn't take too long. There is a whole routine of cleaning out the bowels so the doctors can see what's there. I was told not to drink or eat anything red or purple before the surgery. I guess that would leave a "stain" in the bowels and the doctors couldn't tell if it was blood or not.

The surgery itself went smoothly and the recovery time was only about a week. I am finally starting to feel better and getting back to normal. I can sit for a long time without issues and overall I have a sense of well-being.

Friday, July 18, 2003

I actually went back to work today -- real work, not just visiting. I didn't do anything too strenuous and took a long lunch break. This was an unofficial day back to work to see how things would go. I knew that I couldn't do a full day's work yet; four or five hours and I had to give in and go home.

Tuesday, July 22, 2003

This was my official return to work day. It was a quiet day. I had no major chores to do, but I did manage to participate in one meeting in the library. It was hard staying awake. I don't know if that was because of my physical condition or the subject of the meeting.

I continued to go to work almost every day. I would skip a half-day here and there because I still was so tired all the time. I just didn't want to believe how much the process of getting chemo would take out of me. I certainly have a new respect for anyone who undergoes major surgery or has a baby.

Wednesday, July 25, 2003

I think today is Day+114. Carla and I celebrated our thirty-second wedding anniversary today. A few months ago I wouldn't have bet the farm on me making it here. Carla got a pair of earrings and I sent flowers to her office. We really didn't do much; it was another quiet day.

I made it out for another bike ride, but today it seemed a lot harder. I guess I have to work to get my muscles back in shape; they haven't had to work this hard for quite a while.

Saturday, August 16, 2003

This is one of the defining days that say I am back to normal and I will beat leukemia. The four of us, Carla, Collett, Brett and I left for Jamaica today. We spent a week on the beach relaxing, swimming in the ocean and just being lazy. I was very careful about what I ate and I didn't drink any alcohol the whole time I was there.

From this point on, things quickly returned to normal. After we got back from vacation, I had to go to Roswell for another bone marrow biopsy. My counts are slowly coming up to be where they should be. I just have to continue doing what I'm doing and get to the five-year mark to beat this thing.

SIX YEARS LATER
Monday, March 17, 2009

Saint Patrick's Day is when I celebrate the anniversary of my getting discharged from Roswell after my stem cell transplant. I didn't do anything special on this day; I enjoyed a quiet day at work, went to the gym after work and had a quiet evening at home. I reflected a little about how lucky I was to be here and that people younger than me didn't survive the treatments they had received at Roswell Park Cancer Institute.

After my first Ride for Roswell in 2003, Carla has joined me on the ride. The last two years, our daughter Collett and one of her friends rode with us. In 2008 we were able to raise $1,100.00 for Roswell.

Carla and I participate in a program called "First Contact" that is run by the Leukemia and Lymphoma Society located at RPCI. From time to time we get a call from Colleen Jones asking one of us (or both of us, once in a while) to contact a person who has either just been diagnosed with, or is starting treatment for leukemia. We attempt to answer their questions, tell them of our experiences and try to give them comfort and hope that they too, will make it through to remission.

SEVEN YEARS LATER
May 2010

I started writing this book in the summer of 2008, hoping that I would have it published by Christmas of that year. Obviously, that didn't happen.

A lot has happened since my original adventure began. My daughter got married and divorced – I think Brett stayed with her until he was sure I was back in good health. Collett has completed her master's degree in elementary reading and education; has her exceptional education certification; and just earned her early childhood certification. She begins teaching full time in the fall.

My wife, Carla has survived breast cancer that was discovered during a routine examination by her doctor. I have survived skin cancer that I somehow managed to get on my right thumb, of all places.

I jokingly tell everyone we are going for the volume discount on cancer treatments.

Routine exams are important. Carla had not had a breast exam in two years. When I was diagnosed with leukemia it was more than three years since I had seen a doctor for a check-up.

On March 17, 2010 I became a seven year cancer survivor. I have been going back to Roswell for my annual checkups and now find that Roswell has become more of a research and teaching hospital than a patient care hospital. A lot of the same people are still there, but many of them have moved to different departments. The last time I visited 5-West, only a handful of the staff were the same that treated me. I am not sure that I would receive the same treatment and attention if I were to be just going there now for treatment.

After my latest visit I began thinking about my diagnosis and treatment. I began to think that, perhaps I never really had leukemia.

I was what was called an "RH" baby back in the days when I was born. My father had a blood type of A+ and my mother was A-, thus I was all mixed up and within a few months of being born, I needed several blood transfusions. I was an anemic child and had to take iron supplements for several years.

In 1987, while visiting Cape Cod, I am fairly sure that I contracted Lyme disease. I noticed the warning symbols of red, round splotches on my arms. But, being a man, I pretty much ignored them; wrote them off as just bug bites. About three months after that I had a bout of Bell's palsy. At the time, a person couldn't be tested for Lyme disease unless they were tested within a few days of contracting it. I had waited too long for the doctors to test me to determine what caused my Bell 's palsy and it was written off as just a natural occurrence. I did some research and found out that Bell 's palsy is a relatively common occurrence.

One of Carla's co-workers had a friend that was diagnosed with leukemia. After undergoing one round of chemotherapy he was able to get a second opinion. It turned out that he never had leukemia and began treatment for an entirely different disease. After hearing other such stories and doing some research on the Internet, I began to suspect that it was Lyme disease that either triggered my leukemia or was mimicking it. During one of my annual visits to Roswell Park I had a discussion about this with Dr. Wetzler. He said it was interesting that I asked about this because they had just begun studies to test for such a thing. They were looking at the kinds of viruses, such as Lyme disease, that may trigger Leukemia, and several other diseases,.

When I went into Roswell I was so overwhelmed by everything that I didn't take time to say, wait, back off, and let me think about this. Things were presented in such a way that I didn't think I had time for a second opinion. I know everyone there was really concerned for my well-being, but they scared me so much I didn't think I had a choice. If you can, get a second opinion before starting any treatment.

REFLECTIONS

I've never been the kind of person that "reflected" on the events in my life, but this experience has changed that. Everyone has heard the saying, "Stop and smell the roses", or flowers, or whatever. I am trying to make an effort to be more patient and flexible, although Carla will probably argue that that's not totally true. When I regress, I simply tell her I'm a work in progress. It took me fifty-two years to get here; it might take a little longer to change.

I mentioned that I was in library school when all of this started. I managed to complete my course work from my hospital bed. I submitted my final group project to my professor via email and sent a copy to my cohort. I managed to get an A for that class. I still don't know if it was because of my superior work or because the professor felt sorry for me. That was the only class I took towards my MLS. I came to the conclusion that I had better things to do with my life. One person from my cohort, Lisa Forrest, visited me while I was in the hospital and she brought me a collection of Snoopy cartoons. I still have that book and consider it one of my prized possessions.

There are two books that have made a difference in my life; "The Power of Now" by Eckhardt Tolle and "Radical Gratitude" by Andrew Bienkowski.

From Tolle, I try to remember that there is only "now" and that I should concentrate on that. I shouldn't fret too much about the past or worry too much about the future. I can't change the past, and although I can prepare for the future, the future will decide what happens to me. He also taught me that in any given situation there are only three possible solutions: accept it, change it, or leave. When I'm in a difficult situation, I try to use those options to my advantage.

From Bienkowksi, I learned to be grateful for what I have and to not covet or want more. I have everything I need: a good and loving wife, a beautiful daughter, a nice house, a functioning car, and a pretty good job. There is nothing I need and I am working very hard to be grateful for where I am right now. There is always someone, somewhere, worse off than I am and I try to remember that. When I get down, I think about all I have and I say to myself, "I am truly grateful for everything and everyone in my life."

Carla and I always said that when we retired, we would like to travel and see the world. Getting leukemia changed that; we are not waiting until we retire. We manage to take two vacations a year. We take one in the spring that Carla plans, and we take our daughter Collett and a friend of her choosing. We have been to Jamaica, Grand Cayman, Cozumel, Costa Rica, Belize, Panama, and a few other, out of the way places. We also made our dream trip to Alaska, but Collett didn't come on that one with us. We made up for that by taking her to Disney World.

In the fall we take our second vacation. This one is for just Carla and me. The destination for this one is my choice. I pretend to plan this one, but Carla inevitably takes over and finishes the job. We have been to the four corners – where Arizona, New Mexico, Utah and Colorado touch – the only place in the U.S. where four states meet; we have seen the painted desert, the petrified forest, we went to the Grand Ole Opry in Nashville, and have seen Elvis' mansion in Graceland. I still want to see Easter Island, Tahiti, Mount Rushmore and the Crazy Horse statue. I don't really have a "bucket list", but there are a few more things I want to see and do before I do "kick the bucket".

For the time being I am still working and looking forward to my retirement. I hope Carla and I have a few more years to travel and enjoy life. No matter what happens, I am very grateful for what I have and even though the trip was a rough one, I am glad I made it.

APPENDIX

ROSWELL PARK CANCER INSTITUTE ELM AND CARLTON STREETS
BUFFALO, NY 14263

PRINCIPAL INVESTIGATOR:_____Maria Baer, MD
PROTOCOL NO.:_____CALG13 19808
TITLE: Phase III Randomized Study of Induction
           Chemotherapy With or Without MDR-Modulation
           With PSC-833 (NSC#648265, IND#41121) Followed
           by Cytogenetic Risk-Adapted Intensification Therapy
           Followed by Immunotherapy With RIL-2
           (NSC#373364, IND#1969) Vs Observation in
           Previously Untreated Patients With AML < 60 Years

Informed Consent Given to Patient Taking Part in an

Investigational Procedure:

You (your child) have been diagnosed with acute myeloid leukemia (AML), a cancer of blood cells. For this reason, we are offering you (your child) the opportunity to take part in a research study (a clinical trial) of a new treatment or drug combination being given in a new way. It is important that you (your child) read and understand several general principles that apply to all who take part in our studies:

I. Taking part in the study is entirely voluntary.

2. You (your child) may withdraw from the study at any time without penalty or loss of any benefits to which you (your child) are otherwise entitled.

3. If you (your child) should decide not to participate in this study, it will not affect your (your child's) care at Roswell Park Cancer Institute now or in the future.

4. If you (your child) want a second opinion we will assist you (your child) in obtaining one if you (your child) so desire.

5. Personal benefit may not result from taking part in the study, but knowledge may be gained that will benefit others.

6. Any significant new findings that relate to your (your child's) treatment will be discussed with you (your child).

INTRODUCTION:

It has been explained to you (your child) that you (your child) have a cancer of blood cells, called Acute Myeloid Leukemia (AML), which cannot be removed by surgery or be adequately controlled with radiation treatment. Chemotherapy is the best treatment option available to you (your child) at this time. The type of chemotherapy that is considered to be the standard form of treatment for your (your child's) cancer consists of a combination of drugs: Daunorubicin, Etoposide, and Ara-C.

STUDY PURPOSE:

You (your child) will initially be treated with the standard combination chemotherapy treatment of Daunorubicin, Etoposide, and Ara-C. Following the first cycle of chemotherapy, if you (your child) attain remission, the next step in your (your child's) treatment will be determined by the results of tests done on your (your child's) bone marrow at the time of your (your child's) diagnosis. These tests reveal whether your (your child's) leukemia cells possess characteristics that enable them to respond favorably to chemotherapy. If so, you (your child) will receive three additional cycles treatment with Ara-C. If your (your child's) leukemia cells do not possess favorable characteristics, you (your child) will receive chemotherapy consisting of Ara-C and Etoposide, followed by a peripheral blood stem cell transplant (PBSCT). If it is not considered feasible for you (your child) to have a PBSCT, you (your child) will be assigned a treatment plan of high-dose chemotherapy cycles that include Ara-C and Etoposide. If you (your child) remain in remission, you (your child) will proceed to the final part of the study that will compare the effects (good and bad) of no further treatment, to treatment with an investigational drug known as Interleukin-2 (IL-2). IL-2 is a type of immunotherapy that may stimulate your (your child's) own immune system to kill any residual leukemia cells. This research is being done to determine which of these treatments is the safest and most effective. The results of this study will be closely correlated with other important laboratory studies. Your (your child's) doctor will discuss each of these laboratory studies with you (your child) and ask you (your child) to sign additional consent forms.

STUDY TARGET AND DURATION:

This study will involve approximately 720 patients nationally. The treatment phase of this study will be approximately 8 months, if you (your child) are able to complete all cycles/courses of treatment. Bone marrow samples will be taken 1 month after completion of treatment then every 4 months for 2 years, then at the discretion of your (your child's) doctor, or if there is a suspicion of recurrence of your (your child's) leukemia. You (your child) will be seen at least every 2 months for blood counts for 2 years, then every 6 months for years 3 and 4, then yearly until 10 years after your (your child's) diagnosis, unless you (your child) have other medical problems which require closer follow-up.

STUDY DESCRIPTION IN DETAIL:

There are three parts to the treatment in this study: 1) Induction Chemotherapy; 2) Intensification Chemotherapy, and, if you (your child) are randomized to receive it, 3) Post-Remission Immunotherapy. Each part is explained in detail as follows.

You (your child) will be admitted to the hospital for all of your (your child's) chemotherapy treatments. After completion of each cycle of chemotherapy, you (your child) will be given antibiotics to help fight infections, and blood and/or platelet transfusions to support your (your child's) blood counts. You (your child) will be discharged from the hospital when your (your child's) blood counts have recovered to adequate levels, you (your child) have recovered from the side effects of chemotherapy, and you (your child) no longer require intravenous antibiotics that need to be given in the hospital.

1) *Induction Chemotherapy:*

These drugs are given by intravenous (IV) infusion through a needle in your (your child) arm, or through a "central line," an IV catheter placed in the large vein under your (your child's) collarbone or in your (your child's) neck. Ara-C will be given by a continuous infusion for 7 days. Daunorubicin is a 30 minute infusion and Etoposide is a 2 hour infusion, each given once a day for 3 days, beginning on the same day as the Ara-C. During treatment, various blood tests and X-rays will be used to monitor your (your child's) physical condition. You (your child) will also be asked to have a bone marrow aspiration and biopsy 14 days after starting your (your child's) treatment, to determine if your (your child's) disease has responded to the chemotherapy and again when your (your child's) blood counts are recovering after chemotherapy. If your (your child's) bone marrow aspirate and biopsy show that you (your child) are in remission and you (your child) have recovered sufficiently from this treatment phase, you (your child) will proceed to Intensification. If, however, your (your child's) bone marrow aspirate and biopsy show remaining leukemia, the chemotherapy treatment will be repeated in a shortened version. In this repeated version, Ara-C is given by continuous infusion for 5 days. The Daunorubicin is a 30-minute infusion and Etoposide is a 2-hour infusion given once each day for 2 days. After completion of this course of chemotherapy, you (your child) will again have a bone marrow aspirate and biopsy to determine your (your child's) disease response. If your (your child's) bone marrow biopsy shows that you (your child) are in remission and you (your child) have recovered sufficiently from this treatment phase, you (your child) will proceed to Intensification. If your (your child's) bone marrow aspiration and biopsy still show leukemia, you (your child) will be taken off this treatment protocol and other treatment options will be offered to you (your child).

2) Intensification Chemotherapy:

The intensification treatment you (your child) receive will be determined by the results of routine tests done at the time of your (your child's) diagnosis. If your (your child's) leukemia cells possess characteristics indicating they may respond favorably to chemotherapy alone, you (your child) will receive 3 additional treatments of Ara-C by IV infusion. The doses of Ara-C used for intensification therapy are substantially higher than those used for the induction treatment, and have been previously shown to be more effective than lower doses to maintain remission. Each intensification treatment consists of Ara-C given over a 3 hour period, every 12 hours, (a total of 6 doses) every other day, approximately every 28 days for 3 cycles.

If your (your child) leukemia cells do not possess characteristics indicating they may respond favorably to chemotherapy alone, you (your child) will receive two more cycles of chemotherapy followed by a peripheral blood stem cell transplant (PBSCT) as intensification treatment. For the first cycle of chemotherapy, you (your child) will receive Ara- C and Etoposide. You (your child) will receive the chemotherapy drug Etoposide IV continuously for 4 days (96 hour infusion). You (your child) will also receive Ara-C IV for 2 hours, twice daily for the same 4 days. Beginning two weeks after starting this chemotherapy, you (your child) will receive the drug G-CSF daily by an injection under the skin. G-CSF helps to produce white blood cell recovery more quickly, and stimulates the release of "stem cells" from your (your child's) bone marrow into your (your child's) circulating blood. These "stem cells" are the cells needed later on for the transplant. When a sufficient number of stem cells have been produced, which is about 3 weeks after your (your child's) chemotherapy was given, you (your child) will have them collected by an outpatient procedure called pheresis. During pheresis, your (your child's) blood is removed through a catheter similar to the one you (your child) had in place for the chemotherapy, and processed through a machine that separates the stem cells from the rest of your (your child's) blood. The stem cells are then collected and the rest of your (your child's) blood is returned to you (your child) through your (your child's) catheter. The collected stem cells are then frozen with a preservative called DMSO, for use during the transplant later. Each collection takes about 5 hours, and you (your child) will be awake and comfortable during that time. You (your child) may expect to have collections at least 2 consecutive days, and up to 5 consecutive days.

The most frequent side effect from the pheresis procedure is a buzzing feeling from the medicine used to stop your (your child's) blood from clotting in the machine. Other side effects include muscle cramps, infection, and bleeding. Once your (your child's) stem cells have been collected and frozen, you (your child) will undergo a number of tests to make sure you (your child) are healthy enough to have a PBSCT. These tests will be scheduled to be performed in the outpatient setting, approximately 14 days prior to your (your child's) anticipated date of admission for the transplant. You (your child) will have at least a 4-week rest between your (your child's) last chemotherapy admission and the date of your (your child's) hospital admission for transplant. The pre-transplant tests include x-rays of your (your child's) heart and lungs, breathing tests, kidney tests, blood tests, and a bone marrow aspirate and biopsy to confine that you (your child) are still in remission. After you (your child) are admitted to the hospital for the transplant, you (your child) will receive the chemotherapy drug busulfan either by mouth or IV. If you (your child) receive busulfan by mouth you (your child) will receive it 4 times a day for 4 days. Each individual dose will consist of approximately 25-50 small pills, which will be packaged, in a smaller number of gelatin capsules. If you (your child) receive busulfan IV, you (your child) will receive it every 6 hours as a 2 hour infusion for 4 days, for a total of 16 doses. Anti-nausea medicines will be given to make sure you (your child) do not vomit this important medication. You (your child) will receive medications to prevent seizures. The day after receiving your (your child's) final dose of busulfan, you (your child) will receive Etoposide IV over 4 hours. After a 2 day rest to allow the chemotherapy to completely leave your (your child's) body, your (your child's) stem cells that were previously collected will be thawed and given to you (your child) IV, much like a blood transfusion is given. On the day of the stem cell infusion, and each day thereafter, you (your child) will again receive the drug G-CSF daily by injection under your (your child's) skin until your (your child's) blood counts have recovered to satisfactory levels.

During your (your child's) time in the hospital you (your child) will be supported with blood and platelet transfusions, antibiotics, and nutritional support in a manner similar to that during your (your child's) previous treatments. After being discharged from the hospital, medication will be prescribed to prevent infections until your (your child's) immune system has recovered satisfactorily. You (your child) will be examined frequently in the outpatient setting until you (your child) no longer require transfusions or medication adjustments. Should you (your child) be unable to undergo PBSCT, you (your child) will receive a course of intensification chemotherapy consisting of Etoposide IV continuously for 4 days (96 hour infusion) and Ara-C IV for 2 hours, twice daily for the same 4 days. Following this, you (your child) will receive Ara-C given over a 3 hour period, every 12 hours, for 3 days (a total of 6 doses), approximately every 28 days for 2 cycles.

3) Post-Remission Immunotherapy:

After your (your child's) blood counts have recovered sufficiently following your (your child's) last chemotherapy or transplant treatment, you (your child) will undergo another bone marrow aspirate and biopsy to confirm that you (your child) are still in remission. Then you (your child) will be randomized to receive either immunotherapy with a series of daily injections of the investigational drug called Interleukin-2 (IL-2), or no further treatment. Randomization is a process used to assign patients to different treatment groups. Neither the doctor nor the patient can choose the group. The statistical office will use a computer to randomly assign patients to either group. By using randomization, the groups will be similar and the treatments patients receive can be compared objectively. You (your child) will have an equal chance of being placed in either group. At this time, it is not known which of the treatments is the safest and most effective. After randomization, you (your child) will receive one of the following treatments:

A)   Standard care with close observation, meaning, with no further therapy, OR

B)   An experimental drug known as IL-2

IL-2 has been shown to stimulate human immune defense mechanisms to kill leukemia cells in the laboratory and in some patients. You (your child), a family member, or a friend will be taught to give a low dose of IL-2 by a daily injection much like a diabetic injects insulin every day. An injection instruction sheet and a calendar will be provided to you (your child).

The timing of the daily IL-2 injections can be determined by your (your child's) preference. For example, bedtime injections may decrease side effects from the drug. Every week we will provide you (your child) with 6 small syringes and needles with your (your child's) dose of IL-2 drawn up. You (your child) will keep the syringes in your refrigerator until you (your child) are ready to use one. At the end of the week, you (your child) will return to the hospital or clinic to pick-up a new supply of IL-2. In addition to the daily low-doses of IL-2, we plan to give you (your child) periodic high doses of IL-2. These doses will be injected for 3 days in a row after you (your child) have completed the first 14 days of low-dose IL-2 injections. The 3 days of high-dose IL-2 will be given after each low dose cycle, for a total of 5 complete cycles. If you (your child) complete the first 3-day high-dose IL-2 without serious side effects, you (your child) will be given a slightly higher dose of IL-2 for the remaining 3- day high-dose sequences. After each 3-day high-dose bolus sequence you (your child) will have 1 rest day during which you (your child) will receive no IL-2. The total length of IL-2 immunotherapy treatments will be 90 days. Because the high-dose IL-2 may have more side effects, you (your child) will receive those doses in the outpatient clinic area rather than at home. A calendar will be provided for you (your child) describing when you (your child) should receive the low and high dose injections, and your (your child's) research nurse will follow your (your child's) scheduling as well as your (your child's) progress closely. Additionally, blood will be drawn at various time points to assess the effects of IL-2.

REQUIRED MEDICAL TESTS:
The following routine tests must be done to make sure that you (your child) are eligible for this study:
- Blood and urine tests
- Chest x-ray
- Bone marrow aspirate and biopsy
- EKG and heart scan

Many of these tests will be repeated during different phases of the study. If you (your child) participate in this Research Study, some of these tests may be done more frequently than if you (your child) were not taking part in this research study.

RISKS AND SIDE EFFECTS:
During the study, you (your child) are at risk for the following side effects. You (your child) should discuss these with your (your child's) physician. There also may be other side effects that we cannot predict. Various medications will be given to lessen these side effects. Many side effects go away shortly after the drugs are stopped, but in some cases side effects can be serious, long lasting, or permanent. You (your child) should make sure that your (your child's) physician is aware of any medications that you (your child) are taking, including vitamin supplements; many of the drugs you (your child) will receive on this protocol could interact with your (your child's) medications.

Patients receiving standard chemotherapy agents:

Very Likely Side Effects:
- Lowered white blood cell count* that may lead to infection
- Lowered platelet count* which may lead to an increase in bruising or bleeding
- Lowered red blood cell count ' or anemia, which may cause tiredness, or shortness of breath
- Discolored urine (pink or red) may occur up to 48 hours after Daunorubicin and DSMO is given. This is not harmful.
- Sensitivity to sunlight
- Mouth pain and/or ulcers in the mouth and throat
- Hair loss, which is usually temporary
- Nausea and vomiting
- Loss of appetite or changes in taste sensation

- Constipation or diarrhea
- Fatigue
- Darkening of the nail beds • Rash or dryness of the skin
- Busulfan in the doses given in this study may very likely cause you (your child) to become infertile (unable to have children), although men may occasionally father children.

When these occur, you (your child) may receive blood or platelet transfusions, antibiotics, and/or a reduction in the amount of chemotherapy given to you (your child).

<u>Less Likely Side Effects</u>:
- Liver inflammation resulting in elevated liver function tests or hepatitis not caused by infection
- Fever or chills
- Peeling, flaking, or darkening of the skin; palms of the hands or soles of the feet may tingle, or become numb, painful, swollen, or red
- Eye irritation or conjunctivitis

- Allergic Reaction: Increased heart rate, wheezing, shortness of breath, nasal stuffiness, sinus congestion, sneezing, watery eyes, and runny nose may occur.
- Headache

Less Likely But Serious Side Effects:

- Chemotherapy drugs can be irritating to the skin if they leak out of the vein, resulting in swelling, redness, pain, or ulceration. Report any burning, stinging, or pain while a drug is being given. If the area of injection becomes red and swollen, notify your (your child's) doctor immediately.
- Heart damage, irregular heart rate, or congestive heart failure
- Inflammation of the lungs causing shortness of breath, usually reversible
- Busulfan in high doses can cause irreversible liver damage that can be fatal
- Neurologic changes including: temporary difficulty or unsteadiness when walking, difficulty in focusing, dizziness and/or lightheadedness, confusion, psychosis, seizures, stupor, coma
- Etoposide can cause a drop in blood pressure (low blood pressure).
- Seizures

Patients receiving G-CSF (all reversible when drug is discontinued):

Very Likely Side Effects:

- Muscle aches and/or bone pain; flu-like symptoms
- Fever
- Pain at the injection site

Less Likely Side Effects:

- Chills
- Nausea or loss of appetite
- Liver inflammation causing increased liver function tests

Less Likely But Serious Side Effects:

- Fluid retention
- Irritation of the lining of the heart, or pericarditis

Patients receiving IL-2

Very Likely Side Effects:
- Aches and soreness in joints (arthritis, arthralgia). Headache, muscle aches, low back pain, drowsiness, weakness, or fatigue
- Rash and/or itching
- Fever

Less Likely Side Effects:
- Diarrhea or constipation
- Nausea and/or vomiting
- Lowered blood counts Fluid retention

Less Likely But Serious Side Effects:
- Blood clots which could result in stroke or heart attack Mental changes such as depression, hallucinations, agitation, moodiness, paranoia, restlessness, decreased sexual drive, forgetfulness, sleepiness, nightmares
- Neurological changes such as weakness, fatigue, slurred speech, blindness, deafness, alteration in taste, confusion, seizures
- Kidney or liver toxicity which is usually reversible
- Irregular heart rate or drop in blood pressure
- Fluid retention in the lungs

- Inflammation of the pancreas or gall bladder
- Thyroid dysfunction

Secondary Malignancy: A number of established chemotherapy agents have an inherent risk of causing another cancer (secondary malignancy). Certain drugs in use today, not currently known to be associated with this risk, may be shown at a later time to result in the development of these secondary malignancies.

Related Studies (Optional Participation)

In addition to the treatment study, the researchers would also like to collect additional samples of your blood if your doctor wishes you to receive the busulfan by IV (not by mouth). These blood tests may help determine if there is a way to predict how your tumor will respond to treatment with busulfan and what side-effects you may experience. We ask that you give approval for these tests to be performed using these samples.

Approximately 2 teaspoons of additional blood would be collected at 5 time points during the intensification therapy: just before you receive busulfan for the first time, just after you receive busulfan for the first time, 2 hours and 15 minutes after the bulsufan infusion is started, 4 hours after it is started, and 6 hours after it is started. You will need to have a separate IV (through a needle in a vein in your arm) for blood samples to be obtained. The blood will then be sent to a CALGB laboratory for analysis.

These tests will not involve the study of cancer genes that can be inherited (passed from parents to children).

I agree that additional blood may be used for the research studies described above.

Yes   No   Patient Initials   Date

Reproductive Risks:

This study may be harmful to unborn babies. You should not become pregnant or father a baby while on this study. Also, you should not nurse your baby while on this study. Women of childbearing age will be required to take a pregnancy test before being allowed to participate in this study. The pregnancy test must be negative before starting this study.

You will be asked to practice an effective method of birth control while you are on this study (such as, oral birth control pills, an IUD, condoms with spermicide or abstinence). In women of childbearing age, birth control should continue for six months after the last treatment to ensure that the drug has cleared from the body. Since interactions with oral birth control pills cannot be ruled out, a "barrier" method of contraception (condom, diaphragm) must be used as well.

To the best of your knowledge, you are not pregnant and do not plan to become pregnant while participating in this study. You have been told to practice a medically accepted method of birth control, which you will discuss with your doctor. Should you become pregnant during the course of this study, you will immediately tell your study doctor and obstetrician. Ask about counseling and more information about preventing pregnancy. Pregnancy tests may be repeated during the course of the study.

Male patients must use an effective method of birth control, such as condoms with spermicide, abstinence or have had a vasectomy, when participating in this study and should continue use of birth control for three months after receiving the last dose of the drug to be sure that the drug has cleared from the body. Males who are receiving treatment should not donate sperm for at least six months after the study is completed. Discuss birth control measures with your doctor.

BENEFITS:
It is unknown if this treatment will benefit you (your child) or not. Possible benefits may include an improvement of your (your child's) cancer. This would result in a reduction in your (your child's) symptoms and improvement in your (your child's) quality of life and increase your (your child's) life expectancy. It is also possible that the investigational treatments may prove to be less effective or even harmful to you (your child). No guarantee of benefit can be made to you (your child) for taking part in this research study. Future patients may benefit from the results and knowledge gained from this study.

VOLUNTARY PARTICIPATION:
Taking part in this study is voluntary. You (your child) may choose not to take part or may leave the study at anytime. Leaving the study will not result in any penalty or loss of benefits to which you (your child) are entitled. However, before deciding to stop participating in the study, we encourage you (your child) to talk with your (your child's) doctor first about such a decision.

ALTERNATIVES:
Other treatments for your (your child's) disease include supportive care only (no treatment, but medications and measures to keep you (your child) comfortable), conventional treatment with other drugs, drug combinations, or possibly other research programs which may be testing new drugs for your (your child's) type of cancer. There is no clear evidence that other treatments are significantly more effective than this treatment. You (your

child) should feel free to discuss your (your child's) disease and your (your child's) treatment options with your (your child's) doctor.

REMOVAL FROM STUDY:
Your (your child's) doctor or the sponsor of the study may stop this treatment at any time. You (your child) are free to stop this treatment at any time. Any significant new finding, beneficial or otherwise, will be told to you (your child) and explained as it relates to your (your child's) treatment. If your (your child's) physician becomes aware of significant side effects related to any study drug during the course of treatment, he or she will provide you (your child) with this information and discuss your (your child's) continued participation in this study with you (your child).

USE OF PROTECTED HEALTH INFORMATION (PHI):
If you (your child) do not authorize the use of Protected Health Information as indicated in the consent form, you (your child) will continue to receive care, but not as a part of this study. For the purpose of this study, your (your child) "health information" refers to biographical information, such as your (your child's) name, address, social security or patient number, medical record number, or other items of information that alone or in combination with other information can be used to identify you (your child), information about your (your child's) health, including past history, treatment, diagnosis, test results and any other information about your (your child's) health or conditions, or relating to payment of charges for medical treatment, found in your (your child's) medical record or in other records maintained by Roswell. You (your child) may also withdraw your (your child's) authorization for us to use your (your child's) data, but you (your child) must do so in writing. Withdrawing your (your child's) authorization will make you (your child) ineligible to participate in the research. (Data that has already been authorized for use and disclosed to the Cancer and leukemia Group B (CALGB) cannot be withdrawn).
The results of clinical tests or therapy performed as part of the research may be included in your (your child's) medical record and may not be able to be removed. Your (your child's) decision not to participate or to withdraw from the study will not involve any penalty or loss of benefits to which you (your child) are entitled and will not affect your (your child's) access to health care here. If you (your child) do decide to withdraw, you must contact Maria Baer, MD in writing and let her know that you (your child) are withdrawing from the study. Her mailing address is

Roswell Park Cancer Institute, Elm & Carlton Streets, Buffalo, New York 14263.

CONFIDENTIALITY:

Study records that identify you (your child) will be kept confidential as required by law. Federal Privacy Regulations provide safeguards for privacy, security and authorized access. Except when required by law or otherwise authorized, you (your child) will not be identified by name, address, telephone number or any other direct personal identifier in study records disclosed outside of Roswell Park Cancer Institute. Unless you (your child) have given authorization, study records disclosed outside of Roswell Park Cancer Institute will identify you (your child) only by a unique code number. The key will be kept secure at RPCI.

In addition to the health care personnel involved in this study, your (your child's) treatment records will be available only to representatives of the Food and Drug Administration (FDA), the Office for Human Research Protection (OHRP), the National Cancer Institute (NCI), the National Institute of Health (NIH), the Institutional Review Board (IRB) at Roswell Park Cancer Institute, other government regulatory agencies as permitted by law, and CALGB. We are also asking for your (your child's) consent to notify your (your child's) referring doctor about your (your child's) participation in this study.

We may analyze and/or compare the results of your (your child's) participation in this study along with the results of others who participate. We may present this information at scientific meetings, or we may publish this information in medical literature. In anything we present or publish, there will be no way to identify you (your child) as an individual. Your (your child's) identity will remain confidential, and your (your child's) records will he used by these authorized representatives only in connection with carrying out their obligations relating to the clinical trial or the study drug. They shall not be used for any other purpose or disclosed to any third party except with your (your child's) permission.

AUTHORIZATION FOR USE OF PROTECTED HEALTH INFORMATION:

By signing this form you (your child) are authorizing the use and disclosure, for research purposes, the following information: your (your child's) name, initials, social security number, medical record number or patient identifier number if necessary, date of birth and/or age, sex, admission and discharge dates, date of surgery and/or treatments, (photographs, biometric identifiers, etc...) and your (your child's) diagnosis. By signing this form you (your child) are allowing the research team and other personnel involved in this study to have access to your (your child's) health information.

As part of the study Maria Baer, MD and the study team will report the results of the study-related laboratory tests and x-rays to CALGB. These would include laboratory tests such as your (your child's) blood counts and tests to measure the function of your (your child's) liver, heart, and kidneys and other tests and (x-rays or scans). In addition, your (your child's) records may be reviewed in order to meet federal or state regulations. Reviewers may include, for example, representatives from the Food and Drug Administration, representatives of CALGB, the Roswell Park Cancer Institute Institutional Review Board, Chiron Corp. (the makers of IL-2), and the Office for Human Research Protections (OHRP). It may also be necessary for an outside pathologist or cytogeneticist to have access to your (your child's) PHI to either confirm your (your child's) diagnosis or assign the appropriate treatment for you (your child).

In addition, your (your child's) medical record may be reviewed if you (your child) have had an adverse event or a reaction to the study drug or treatment. The information surrounding the adverse event or reaction may be released to CALGB, the FDA, NCI, NIH, and the IRB. PHI may be disclosed without your (your child's) authorization to a person subject to the jurisdiction of the FDA if the drug, device, product or study is governed by the FDA. PHI may be used and disclosed to gather information on the safety, effectiveness, and during analysis of the study. PHI may also be used in the creation and maintenance of a research database or research repository and be kept indefinitely.

This authorization will not expire. Any research information that is part of your (your child's) medical record will be kept indefinitely. You (your child) have the right to see the research related information that is also a part of your (your child's) medical record after the research is completed. However, information obtained in the course of the research will not be shared with you (your child) while the research is being conducted. By signing this form you (your child) are temporarily waiving your (your child's) right to see this information. If you (your child) have questions about this authorization or your (your child's) rights under the privacy law, please contact the Privacy Officer at (716) 845- 5990.

This information may be further disclosed by CALGB, the FDA, the Nth, or the NCI. If disclosed by the sponsor, the information is no longer covered by the federal privacy regulations. RPCI is not responsible for re-disclosures that may occur by a third party. In the event that you (your child) should die while enrolled in or after participation in this study, PHI may be used or disclosed solely for research purposes without obtaining any additional authorization.

AUTHORIZATION:
As a participant in this study, I authorize the use of protected health information for research purposes as indicated above. I understand that PHI will he used only as authorized. I also understand that I have the right to withdraw my authorization for use of PHI, in writing, but that information used or disclosed before my written withdrawal will continue to be used for research purposes. Finally, I understand that persons receiving my PHI through my authorization may further disclose it without the benefit of federal privacy protections.

COSTS:
You (your child) will receive no payment for taking part in this study. The laboratory testing, x-ray and scanning procedures and physicians charges you (your child) will incur as a participant in this study are considered standard of care, and therefore will be your responsibility or that of your third party payer (medical insurance). You will be responsible for all co-

payments and deductibles as required by your individual insurance carrier. _Costs will be billed to you or your insurer in the ordinary manner. Procedures such as x-rays, scans, and laboratory tests purely related to the research and not required for your (your child's) care will not be charged to you. The standard chemotherapy drugs used in this study are approved for the treatment of your (your child's) disease and commercially available medications; you or your insurance carrier will be responsible for the costs of this medication. RIL-2 is an investigational drug and will be provided free of charge by the Division of Cancer Treatment, and the National Cancer Institute (NCI).

In addition, the use of medications to control side effects could result in added costs. Either you or your insurance company will be responsible for the costs of these drugs. In some cases, third party carriers (insurance companies, health care plans, Medicare, Medicaid) may not cover these costs. In the event of complications, you or your health insurance will be billed for the cost(s) of the usual and customary medical care. Neither the sponsor (CALGB), the investigator, nor Roswell Park Cancer Institute will make any payment for injury or complications resulting from your (your child) being in this research project. If you (your child) are injured from this research activity, medical treatment will be provided. Information concerning the policies in this regard or information about the conduct of this study may be obtained from your (your child's) physician.

COMPENSATION:
Roswell Park Cancer Institute will provide short-term medical care for any injury resulting from your (your child's) participation in a research study here. Nothing herein shall obligate Roswell Park Cancer Institute or the State of New York to provide financial compensation or long-teen medical, emotional or psychological treatment for injuries associated with research. It is possible that this research project will result in the development of beneficial treatments, devices, new drugs, or possible procedures.

In this event, you (your child) understand that you (your child) cannot expect to receive any financial compensation from the subsequent use of information acquired and developed through your (your child's) participation in the research project. Your (your child's) agreement of these conditions does not constitute a waiver of any rights you (your child) have under federal or state laws and regulations.

QUESTIONS:

You (your child) should ask your (your child's) doctor any questions you (your child) have about this study. We will fully discuss any questions that you (your child) have about taking part in this study, now or at any later time. You (your child) may direct any questions about this study to Dr. Maria Baer at Roswell Park Cancer Institute, Elm & Carlton Streets, Buffalo, NY, 14263. You may telephone her at (716) 845-7610. In case of an emergency after regular hospital hours, you may call the Department of Medicine Doctor-On-Call at (716) 845-2300. You should direct any questions about research subjects' rights or questions about injury to the Patient Advocate at (716) 845-4474.

ADDITIONAL INFORMATION:

You (your child) may call the NCI's Cancer Information Service at: 1-800-4—CANCER (1-800-422--6237) or via TTY: 1-800-332-8615. You (your child) may visit the NCI's Web sites at: cancer trials: comprehensive clinical trials information htth://caneertrials.nci.nih.gov. CancerNet™: accurate cancer information including PDQ http://cancernet.nei.nih.gov

Cancer Fax: Includes NCI information about cancer treatment, screening, prevention, and supportive care. To obtain a contents list, dial 301/402-5874 or 800/624-2511 from a fax machine hand set and follow the recorded instructions. Additional information about the drugs used in this study is listed on the Medscape web site: www.medscape.com.

PATIENT'S STATEMENT OF CONSENT:

By signing below, you (your child) agree that:

You have (your child has) been told of the reasons for this study.

- You have (your child has) had the study explained to you.
- You have (your child has) had all of your questions answered, including those concerning areas your child) did not understand, to your satisfaction.
- You have (your child has) carefully read this consent form and will receive a copy of this signed form.
- You willingly give your consent (for your child) to voluntarily join in this research study.

PATIENT SIGNATURE

*Printed Patient Name*_____DATE_____TIME_____

ASSENT STATEMENT: N/A

(Where child in the opinion of the treating physician understands enough to give consent and can signify the information in the above study was described to the child participant. The child's signature below indicates his/her assent to participate in this study.

CHILD SIGNATURE_____DATE_____TIME_____

Printed Name of Child _

OR: (If the child cannot read and oral assent is obtained from the child)

The information in the above consent was described to my child and my child verbally agrees to participate in the study.

PARENT/GUARDIAN SIGNATURE_____DATE_____TIME_____

Printed Name of Parent/Guardian

_____

INVESTIGATOR'S STATEMENT:

I certify that to the best of my knowledge the subject/guardian signing this consent form had the research fully and carefully explained to him/her, and I believe clearly understands the nature, risks, and benefits of participation.

www.ingramcontent.com/pod-product-compliance
Lightning Source LLC
Chambersburg PA
CBHW072200280526
45788CB00002B/806

* 9 7 8 1 4 5 2 8 7 2 1 8 6 *